The Book on Immediate Self Defense

Practical Strategies for Everyone

Tony Johnson

THE BOOK ON IMMEDIATE SELF DEFENSE
Practical Strategies for Everyone

Published by
10-10-10 Publishing
Markham, Ontario
CANADA

ISBN-13: 978-1530058693

For information about special discounts for bulk purchases, please
contact 10-10-10 Publishing at 1-888-504-6257
Printed in the United States of America

Contents

DEDICATION

I dedicate this book to my Why:
Myrna, Leslie, and Jessica

TESTIMONIALS

"Tony, when I heard you were writing a book on Self Defense, I was very excited for you. I know it's going to be amazing, and I hope it will help you get even more recognition for all the work you do, you deserve it. You've been teaching Self Defense here in our community to many different groups on an ongoing basis for years now. At Sonoma State University, for Real Estate and other specialty interest groups, at our National Night Out event in cooperation with the Department of Public Safety (Police and Fire), at businesses, and to our community members in general. All I hear are good things. Last year you and the non-profit school you founded were honored for service to our city. It's been a pleasure getting to know you through Rotary, and on behalf of the City of Rohnert Park, congratulations on your book!"
Gina Belforte, Mayor, City of Rohnert Park

"Tony has visited my Freshman Interest Group (FIG) class at Sonoma State University for the past few years. Has talked to my students about risks to personal safety that are present on campus and in the surrounding Rohnert Park community. He engaged the students in conversation about his personal experiences as well as theirs, opening their eyes to the need to be aware and prepared for unexpected circumstances. He then led the class in performing simple, effective responses to use if they found themselves in an unsafe situation. Tony had a great presence with the students, many of which originally did not plan on participating, but were drawn into the activities under Tony's guidance. I believe that the personal safety skills that Tony taught to my students are very important and should be taught to all incoming freshman. "
Jacquelyn Guilford, PhD, Sonoma State University

"Having 13 years of gymnastics under my belt I have experienced a few injuries, which have in turn helped me to raise my body awareness. Because of my unique experience it has been difficult to find individuals who share similar knowledge and understanding of proper posture and safe movement, Tony is one of the few people who not only understands this but also strongly enforces it. Tony is an expert in his field and he demonstrates this not only in his multiple certifications and awards but in his everyday classes. With his extensive knowledge in biomechanics and Martial Arts he is a leader in teaching safe and effective self-defense, Martial Arts, and kickboxing exercises to anyone interested and willing to learn. Tony has developed a strong welcoming environment within his class settings as a result of integrating proper sports etiquette into his teachings. His passion for what he teaches and his expertise in Martial Arts make Tony an inspiring teacher and leader."
Tanisha Larsen, Sonoma State University, Student Coordinator for InMotion

"Sensei Tony taught a very informative, fun self-defense class for over 300 sorority women at Panhellenic's 3rd Annual Women's Wellness Retreat. Numerous women came up to me and told me how great they thought his class was and how they want to continue to learn more about Self Defense and Martial Arts. Tony is not only a great teacher, but a kind individual who wants to spread the importance of self-defense among college women."
Melissa Welch, Panhellenic Executive Board, SSU

"Tony is a very engaging speaker and a highly capable instructor… and a really nice guy who genuinely cares about people being safe and feeling safe."
Diane Novak, North Bay Association of Realtors

"Sensei Tony Johnson is a very valuable part of our Northern California Karate Federation, and has become a good friend. He is very active in serving his community, and exemplifies the true spirit of Karate-Do. I'm so excited for him on the release of his new book, and I look forward to reading it."

Alex Miladi
7th Degree Black Belt: SKUSA, JKA, ISKS
Karate Referee: USAK (USA Karate), PKF (Pan-American Karate Federation), WKF (World Karate Federation)
Vice President/Technical Director : SKUSA (Shotokan Karate USA)
President: NCKF (Northern California Karate-do Federation)
Referee Director: Board of Directors: USAK (USA Karate)

"I'm proud to celebrate the release of The Book on Immediate Self Defense with my friend, Sensei Tony Johnson. He is a real asset to our Regional and National Karate organizations, and dedicated to lifelong learning. I have been able to offer many trainings with top level international athletes and teachers, and Tony comes at every opportunity. He is dedicated to continuous improvement, ongoing training, and lifelong learning. He is always active in serving his community. He sets an example we should all follow."

Sensei Mary Crawford
Chief Instructor/Owner Okaigan Karate International
Northern California Karate Federation Chief Referee
USA National Karate Federation AA Referee
Pan American Karate Federation AA Referee
World Karate Federation AA Referee

"We are lifelong friends. When my brother and I introduced him to Aikido, we never imagined Martial Arts would become the focus of his life. At least not at first. I quickly realized he was serious when he and I started our own practice sessions that involved a lot of, well, get on the mat and fight, let see what techniques we can pull off. Those were always fun, and a lot of good lessons were learned. Many times painfully. A few years ago I had the opportunity to watch him teach a seminar, it was the first time I had ever seen him teach, and I was impressed with how good of an instructor he had become. His book will be a great addition to any serious martial artist library. Congratulations Tony!"
Casey Rodgers

"I appreciate, especially, the non-intimidating environment and interaction. Thank you. I realize it's a true need in our community, and a blessing you are here to fill it."
Michelle Martin, Primerica

"Please let this letter confirm that Tony Johnson, with Immediate Self Defense at Martial Arts Academy, performed a Self Defense Class for Colleagues of the Fairmont Sonoma Mission Inn & Spa. He was very professional and provided valuable information for our colleagues as part of our Health and Safety program which allowed them to feel more secure on property while performing their job duties."
Kaitlyn Tinder, Assistant Director of Human Resources
The Fairmont Sonoma Mission Inn & Spa

"We would like to thank you for your support and participation in our first annual Campus Safety Week during the week of October 13 through October 16, 2014. Your participation allowed us to enhance the safety of our campus community. Through our combined efforts, we were able to interact with more than 1,000 members of the campus community by presenting various topics, such as general safety awareness, sexual assault prevention, alcohol awareness and disaster preparedness. Your time and commitment were greatly appreciated and will undoubtedly make a difference in the community we collectively serve. Thank you again for your support, and we look forward to working with you again next year."
Nathan Johnson, Ed. D. Police Chief & Executive Director
Office of Police and Safety Services

"I would like to wholeheartedly recommend Tony Johnson as a public speaker for any group or event interested in self-defense. In September 2014, a female Real Estate agent in Arkansas was tragically murdered while showing a home to a stranger. In the aftermath of this terrible event, I reached out to Tony to see if he would be willing to address our local group of real estate professionals. Not only was Tony willing to speak to our group, he also donated his time and studio to sponsor a FREE one hour "Safety Awareness and Self-Defense" class. Tony's presentation was excellent! His in depth knowledge of Self Defense combined with his common sense approach to communicating the ideas to our group made for a very interesting presentation. In less than 30 minutes Tony was able to convey many simple but effective self-defense ideas to our group of business men and women. Everyone in the room was captivated by his presentation and the Q & A afterwards elicited many questions along with sharing of many personal experiences. If you are looking for a knowledgeable, well prepared and entertaining speaker, I strongly encourage you to call Tony Johnson."
Tim Carroll, CMG Financial

"Over the past 30 years, I've had the opportunity to study under some great and not-so-great instructors, in a fairly broad range of martial art styles. Sensei Tony is definitely in the 'great' category. Sensei Tony embodies the full range of aspects required to fully study Martial Arts. Not only does he exhibit superb physical skills, but his background knowledge of the origins, specifics and ideals of the Martial Arts is impressive. His commitment to the community is legend, and his commitment to his students is excellent. I heartily recommend Sensei Tony to anyone wanting to really get a 'full immersion' into Martial Arts."
Bill Conde

"Going into detail of the why behind techniques is helpful. It has made me a more friendly person when in uncomfortable situations, rather than being simply worried."
Alexa Chipman

"I appreciated the time Tony took to answer questions during the lessons and how he would immediately implement them into the lesson for everyone to learn. I learned a tremendous amount and had a fun time as well."
Leandra Neely

"Easy to pick up. Friendly environment. Clear instruction. Concepts flow well together."
Amanda Mantynen

"I wanted to personally Thank You for giving that talk this morning and sharing some experiences. Especially since I know first-hand how a little information can save someone's life, it did mine and that is a fact. And I learned just from taking my kids to karate/Self Defense classes and sitting and watching them. Our phone has been ringing a lot this morning, even Realtors signing up their wives. It so important and so necessary. Thank you for all you do to help keep us all safe."
Karla Huffman, CMG Financial, on my talk at the NORBAR (North Bay Association of Realtors) meeting.

"I have attended Martial Arts Academy in Rohnert Park since February of 2013. I have had the opportunity to train at over five schools across the country through my nine years of training in the Martial Arts. Martial Arts Academy is by far my favorite school and our Sensei Tony Johnson is an incredibly skilled and thoughtful instructor. As an educator I can appreciate the varied approaches to his teaching style, and it is clear he reaches each student where they are and helps them improve and create a community. I have taken kickboxing and kung fu classes as well as private lessons and they have been of an exceptional value to me. The classes have provided stress relief, an outlet for pregnancy fitness and an opportunity to make friends and become a part of wonderful community."
Sami Lange, Second Degree Black Belt, Tae Kwon Do

"I have taken several Self Defense classes from Sensei Tony. He is an excellent instructor who works well with all skill levels to teach practical skills for keeping yourself and your loved ones safe. I highly recommend this class."
Janet Henker

"On behalf of the students and staff of John Reed Elementary School we wish to thank you and your students at the Martial Arts Academy Bujutsu Gakuin Wushu Xueyuan (a non-profit corporation) for providing our students with a Lion Dance demonstration and performance. Our children were in awe of the dance and information you presented. It is wonderful community members like yourself that make our school such a wonderful place to learn. We appreciate the time you took to explain and describe the history and culture to our students."
Susan Lopez, Principal, John Reed Elementary School

"Thanks again for your amazing presentations today! Here's a testimonial, feel free to use it in any publication/website, you have my complete endorsement! Sensei Tony Johnson has donated over 12 hours of karate classes for the students in the CalSERVES after-school programs at 6 elementary schools in the Wright and Bellevue School districts of Santa Rosa. As the volunteer coordinator at one of those sites, I really appreciated his approach to teaching students the basics of karate. He was assertive, kind, and demonstrated an amazing ability to captivate students with his contagious enthusiasm. The students not only learned key points in the art of karate, but also got in great physical workouts and were empowered through his presentation. I would highly recommend Sensei Tony for both youth and adults who are interested in learning the karate ABCs, or for advanced lessons. We can't wait to have him return!
Richelle Andrae, CalSERVES AmeriCorps Volunteer Coordinator at Taylor Mountain School

"My name is Julianna Whittaker, and I am the volunteer coordinator for CalSERVES, at Bellevue Elementary School. We are a not-for-profit educational after school program set up in South West Santa Rosa. We always look for ways to involve the community and present different opportunities for the kids during the after school program. Recently, we had Tony Johnson come and present on the art of Karate. He visited us from the Martial Arts Academy at Callinan Sports and Fitness Center in Rohnert Park. He conducted a 25 min presentation to kids divided up in 3 different groups. The groups consisted of K-1st grade, 2-3rd grade, and 4-5-6th grade. He was able to keep the children entertained and held their attention very well. The kids were able to gain positive knowledge of Karate, and were even able to mirror moves that they learned during the presentation. I would highly recommend Tony Johnson's Martial Arts Academy to present in schools because of his dedication to Karate, and his great way of keeping the kids involved and at attention. The kids were clearly enjoying the activity and all asked when he was coming back."
Julianna Whittaker, CalSERVES VIP at Bellevue Elementary

"My name is Lauren Loeffler. I am the CalSERVES Volunteer Coordinator at Wright Charter School. CalSERVES is an AmeriCorps program operating in six different Santa Rosa schools. During the day, we offer one-on-one tutoring for students struggling in their regular curriculum. After school, we provide extra enrichment activities for an additional 150 students. Though we focus mainly on literacy and homework help, our students are also exposed to P.E., science, art, and nutrition. We invited Tony Johnson to our school because he was able to introduce our kids to a new and different sport. Generally, the students at Wright are involved in common sports, such as soccer, basketball, and football. In keeping with our values, Tony had fun with the first through fourth graders and got them moving around. Most importantly however, Tony taught them that Karate is the last resort--safety always comes first. The kids at Wright adored their time with Tony. The students who didn't get to see his presentation are eager for his next visit. I recommend his classes to any family looking to get their child into this discipline. On a personal note, I am excited to participate in his adult kickboxing class. Tony offers something for all ages. I hope that everyone checks out their opportunities!"
Lauren Loeffler, CalSERVES VIP Fellow at Wright Charter School

"My name is Melissa Collins, and I am a team leader at CalSERVES Kawana Elementary. We are a volunteer based after-school program that serves southwest Santa Rosa. We are constantly looking for ways to broaden the kids' horizons and expand their world experiences. Tony Johnson came in and provided an interactive Karate experience. He visited us from the Martial Arts Academy at Callinan Sports and Fitness Center in Rohnert Park. Tony presented to three different groups ranging from K-5. The kids had been reading about karate the week before so the excitement was running high. They absolutely loved his hands on presentation and felt inspired afterwards to continue their Karate education. I would definitely recommend Tony Johnson's Martial Arts Academy to present in schools because he kept the kids involved, made sure to set safety boundaries, and it was appropriate for all age groups (4 through 11). Just today the kids were asking me when that super cool karate man was coming back."
Melissa Collins, Team Leader at CalSERVES Kawana Elementary

Proclamation

A Proclamation of the City Council of the City of Rohnert Park

Recognizing Tony Johnson and Martial Arts Academy
武術学院 Bujutsu Gakuin Wushu Xueyuan
for Service to the City of Rohnert Park

Whereas, the City of Rohnert Park is dedicated to promoting the health, fitness, and cultural enrichment of all of its residents;

Whereas, training in the martial arts has long been recognized as providing superior benefits for the mind, body, and spirit for people of all ages;

Whereas, the purpose of martial arts is to empower practitioners to overcome weaknesses and develop into strong-minded, healthy citizens that can be of benefit to the community;

Whereas, Martial Arts Academy teaches practitioners to respect oneself, to respect others, to do our best, to never give up, and to always remember that martial arts is used for self-defense only; values we can all respect; and

Whereas, Martial Arts Academy is dedicated to accepting all interested students, regardless of financial ability in keeping with its mission which is to "Share the benefits of Martial Arts with Everyone."

Now, Therefore, be it Proclaimed that I, Amy O. Ahanotu, as Mayor and on behalf of the City Council of the City of Rohnert Park, do hereby offer our thanks to Tony Johnson and *Martial Arts Academy 武術学院 Bujutsu Gakuin Wushu Xueyuan* for service to Rohnert Park residents and commend your dedication to enriching our community.

Duly and Regularly Proclaimed this 10th day of February, 2015.

CITY OF ROHNERT PARK

Amy O. Ahanotu, MAYOR

ACKNOWLEDGEMENTS

First I would like to thank my wife Myrna. Without her, I would not be the person I am today. From the beginning, she's seen greatness in me, and helped me rise to meet my destiny. Everyone says that she's the best thing that has ever happened to me, because it's true. I'd like to thank Leslie, Jessica, and Myrna, my Why.

I'd like to thank my family, all of you, for your help and support through all of life's ups and downs. I'd like to thank my mother, who always imagined me for great things, when I did not see them in myself. I know you can see me from Heaven, and that you are guiding me every day. I'd like to thank my father. It was so great to reconnect with you and spend time with you recently, more time than we've spent in more than 20 years. I'd like to thank my sisters, my first best friends. Seeing you and your families for the holidays was so uplifting.

I'd like to thank my teacher, Sensei/Sifu Tim McFarland, and all my Martial Arts Teachers and Mentors for showing me the way, and teaching me all I know. I will faithfully transmit everything I can. Thank you to all teachers I know, for your example, your advice, your guidance, your camaraderie, your vision, and your friendship. I'd like to thank all my students, past, present, and future, without you, the purpose of my life could not be fulfilled. Know that I learn as much from each of you, as you could ever learn from me. It is my great privilege to know you, and serve you.

I'd like to thank all my martial brothers & sisters, but especially Sensei Casey Rodgers, Logan Rodgers, Sensei Chris Field, Reid Andersson, Sifu Jim Suits, Sifu Aaron Beatty, Sensei David Jackson, and Sensei Ed McMillen, some of the greatest partners, seniors, and friends I've ever had the privilege to train with. I'd like to thank Steve Brumme, who embodies the ideals of a warrior, for his example and inspiration.

I'd like to thank the board of directors of the non-profit I founded, John Sciamanna, Ron Evans, and Marian Van Horn. It is because of your support that I feel empowered in our non-profit. I am so grateful for all the help and support from Beverly, Susan, Omar, Raquel, Lisa, Bryan, and so many of my students and their parents who help so much to make it all happen for our school. You guys are amazing; I couldn't do it without you!

I'd like to thank the leadership of Sonoma State University, and all my friends there, who have helped me in immeasurable ways. Especially Cecilia & Dan O'Brien, Marian Van Horn, Nicole Hendry, Janet Henker, Mo Phillips, Chief Nathan Johnson, Officer Eric Wilde, Ryan Fitzpatrick, and so many more.

I'd like to thank all my friends with the City of Rohnert Park, Mayor Gina Belforte, our previous mayor Amy Ahanotu, retired Recreation Director Guy Miller, Community Services Manager Mitch Austin, Community Services Supervisor Nelle Herman, Community Services Program Coordinator Chris Morgan, General Services Supervisor Tom Kelley, City Manager Darrin Jenkins, Assistant City Manager Don Schwartz, Community Development Assistant Suzie Azevedo, Director of Public Works & Community Services John McArthur, Fire Marshal Dan Adams, and many more.

I'd like to take a moment for special thanks to Chief of Police of Rohnert Park, Director of Public Safety, Brian Masterson who took his valuable time and spoke to me at length, ensuring that I had the best info for my book. I'd also like to thank Retired Chief of Police of Cotati, Bob Stewart, who took the time to meet with me and give me the benefit of his perspective and experience.

I'd like to thank the Rotary Club of Rohnert Park/Cotati, and all my friends there. You do so much to help in our community! I am proud to be a member.

I'd like to thank Adam Markel, Michael Silvers, Hawk, Aaron Huey, and everyone at New Peaks. You are doing tremendously important work, and I'm proud to be involved. Your introduction to Raymond Aaron was invaluable, and I've met so many amazing mentors and peers through your organization. Keep up the good work, and I will see you soon. I'd like to thank Nick Vujicic, the very embodiment of positivity and how to thrive in spite of circumstances most of us could not imagine.

Despite this huge list of people to thank, it is hardly comprehensive. I have had help from so many people; I really cannot list them all. Thank you, each and every one. All of you have had a tremendous impact on the book – and your help and support has been so valuable!

Every book I've read, every lecture, workshop, and class I've attended, you've added to my understanding and perspective. Every lecture I've given, every class and workshop I've taught, they've all helped me to get to this point in my journey, and have allowed me to serve you at this level.

Thank you, dear reader. My efforts have been to serve you. Any mistakes, omissions, or missteps are entirely my own. I hope that you can take the best and discard the rest. Your feedback is greatly appreciated.

Lastly, I'd like to thank my Book Architect, Naval Kumar, and my Author/Mentor Raymond Aaron for all their help in making this book better than I ever could have made it on my own. You made this dream come true!

FOREWORD

Have you ever considered how your life and the lives of the ones you love would change if you were assaulted by a criminal and did not know how to defend yourself? You might think it will never happen to you, but the statistics prove that no matter where you live in the world, no matter what you look like, chances are, you WILL someday face a criminal.

What holds you back from learning what you need to know? Is it that you think the subject is too complicated? Good News! Tony has found a way to completely demystify Self Defense, and make it appropriate and reasonable for you to learn, and this book is a great way to get started.

Maybe, instead, you think that learning Self Defense will cost too much? You need to read this book! The book is not expensive, and it could literally save your life. If you want to continue your training, Tony offers advice on exactly how to do that, with him, and even how to find the right local professional.

You might be concerned that learning Self Defense will take too long. Immediate Self Defense will revolutionize the way that Self Defense is taught, making it easier and quicker to teach these essential concepts than ever before. Instead of complicated memorization, Immediate Self Defense is natural, automatic, and already part of your nervous system. There is NO faster way to learn these concepts.

I'm very excited to see this book get published. Self Defense is an important subject, and this book is fun, approachable reading on what could be a challenging subject. In reviewing the book, I was shocked at how many people and organizations in his community endorse Tony and love his live training events. Tony has really made an impact in his community, and now he is starting to do live training events in other locations! I'm proud to help Tony to springboard his Self Defense career to the next level, and so proud of his efforts with this book.

Raymond Aaron
NY Times Bestselling Author

Chapter 1
Introduction

Who is this book for?

This book is written for the average person. The person who has huge gaps in awareness and habits that could draw a criminal to choose you as a target for a crime. This book is for college students, who are particularly vulnerable (at least 1 in 5 will be assaulted while they are in college). This book is for women, who are more frequently victims of criminal assault. This book is for parents, men and women, so they can learn what they need to know to protect themselves, their families, and their children.

This book is for people who would love to learn Self Defense, but thought they didn't have the time or money to learn, or felt the subject was too complicated. It's my mission to completely demystify self-defense. I want the skills and mindset to be easily accessible to you.

I have a confession to make, though. You can't learn physical Self Defense through a book. For that, I would need to show you in a more in depth way than I can through a couple pictures. I created www.immediateselfdefense.com to be a way to connect people with these life-saving skills long distance. Also, I will be doing workshops in different places; please join my mailing list, and I'd love to meet you in person and teach you these skills first-hand.

If you want to find a program closer to you, a section of the book talks about how to find a good program in your area, and what to look for in a class. Another section talks about Martial Arts, in case you are interested in learning more.

If you are a Martial Arts or Self Defense teacher, and you like what you see and would like to implement my methods in your own programs, please connect with me, as I would like to license qualified instructors in Immediate Self Defense. (See the last chapter for more info).

This book is for anyone who has ever had an interest in Self Defense, and wants to learn the right way. This book is for everyone who NEVER had an interest in Self Defense, but suddenly realizes that they should probably learn. There are a lot of things happening these days that make people realize that maybe it's time to learn.

This book is NOT for law enforcement or military personnel. They should hopefully already have been trained in concepts far beyond what the average person would need. Law enforcement also has to work within restrictions that average citizens don't have to worry about at all. Military personnel frequently operate in active zones that require a completely different mentality than one that is appropriate for civilians in Self Defense situations. There are very special considerations in those fields that you, the average civilian, does not need.

This book is also not written for Martial Arts experts, though the concepts that you will be exposed to through this book should already be part of all Martial Arts study. If you are a martial artist or Martial Arts teacher, I should mention that my favorite part of Martial Arts is the practical application of ancient forms. I have an incredible teacher who focuses on the practical, and I have had amazing mentors who have helped me to unlock the secrets hidden away in all the forms I know. If this is something that you are interested in, functional forms training, you should contact me, and let's reinvigorate your practice of the forms. Amazing drills are preserved in those forms that the ancient masters thought was so important, and human biology has not changed in all that time.

This book will make the biggest impact to people who are totally unprepared to handle a Self Defense situation. Strategies you will learn will give you a huge edge, and prepare you to survive a confrontation with a criminal.

In short, this book is for you. All of you, and everyone you care about.

What this book is NOT

This book is NOT a substitute for physical training. A book cannot address physical defense much, as you cannot get the hands-on feeling by simply reading. There can BE no substitute for physical training. It is too important. Words are just words, but taking physical actions will make you capture the feelings of the motions and strategies, and help you understand their importance. You will need to take a class, probably every year or two, to keep these skills sharp and accessible so that you can use them should you ever need them. With enough practice, all the skills become natural and automatic.

I have done many lectures on Self Defense, and I know that many people will never take a physical class. Often the people who have a higher-priority need to learn Self Defense will attend a lecture or read a book, but never step foot in a class. I wish it wasn't true, but I see it all the time. Sometimes I see those same people who attended a lecture but not a physical class the first time around later on. After a couple years I see them again and they finally take my physical class, and they often tell me privately that they suffered an assault and want to make sure they are better prepared in case it ever happens again. Sometimes they are too embarrassed to come to a class, but they call or write me to say how they wish they had taken the physical class and what a difference it could have made in their life.

No book can be a substitute for physical training, but because most crimes are crimes of opportunity, you can learn what makes you attractive to a criminal, and avoid those behaviors which increase your chances of being a target. I have a section of the book devoted to this. For people who will not do physical training, I want to give you the most important concepts that I can, and let you know that there are classes out there where you can feel comfortable, and learn what you really need to know. However, no one can do it for you, you have to decide that you are a valuable person, and that you have a right to survive and live in peace.

This book is not going to do the work for you. You will have to read it and apply the messages. You will have to be willing to look at your habits objectively and take the steps necessary to improve your habits to remove yourself as a target.

This book cannot get you in shape. If you are in terrible physical condition, you are a bigger target for a criminal, and no book can help you get fit. That will require you to value yourself and take the steps necessary to eat healthy and get regular exercise. I encourage you, if you want to start a new exercise routine, to spend the money to get a personal trainer to get started, as well as joining a fun group (aerobics, interval training, Martial Arts, anything that gets your heart rate up and gets you sweating). If you spend the money and get a trainer, you have an appointment, and it is painful and expensive to miss. This is very motivating to most people. Kaiser and many other hospital organizations also offer long-term plans (some even 18 months), that can totally help you change all your health habits, and improve your life. Aren't you worth it? Don't you want to be there for your family?

This book cannot show you what you need to know to defend yourself physically. Pictures really wouldn't do it. For that, the best thing to do is to learn in person. I do lectures, workshops, and hands-on trainings; join our mailing list and let's see if I can come to your area. If training in person with me is not possible, I have a section of the book on how to identify a good program; hopefully you can find one in your area. The physical skills can also be learned by video on my website, www.immediateselfdefense.com

The biggest reason that I teach Self Defense is because of the enormous difference it can make in your life. Knowing how to defend yourself could actually be the difference between life and death. I got into Martial Arts because I was interested in Self Defense. I had been bullied, and I had been able to make it through those situations, but not because of any skill, only through anger, a will to survive, and through sheer meanness. In the animal kingdom, it is entirely different if you are fighting for your life versus fighting for your dinner. It is the same for people.

I think those early experiences of Self Defense made an impression on me. I wanted to feel safe, but I didn't want to be mean, cruel, or have to do terrible things to people to defend myself. I had hurt people who were trying to hurt me, and I felt bad. I had lost friends over bad situations. So I moved away from my original interest in Self Defense, and there came a time when I was more into some of the flashier aspects of Martial Arts: demonstrations, performances, and tournament competition (fighting with rules is totally different than Self Defense). I was a young teacher, and seduced by the flash of the fancy moves, however impractical in real life. All of that was a lot of fun for me and I really enjoyed it, and because I had skill and knowledge, I didn't need to defend myself physically anymore. I knew what to do, and avoided bad situations. If something did happen, I could take care of it easily, so it was no longer a concern. Perhaps I was having my students focus more on these other areas too, but we always did some Self Defense along the way, thank goodness.

Then everything changed. Within a couple months, I had heard from several of my students how they had defended themselves, and how the skills I had taught them had made a huge difference in their lives. They were all great stories, and I was very happy to have had that impact, and helped them stay safe. One story in particular really hit hard, because it happened to a longtime student, and it could have easily ended up a horror story.

This student was a young teenager, very petite, who was doing everything that we would advise not to do (and me and probably many of you have done exactly the same thing many times). She was walking alone, late at night, in near darkness, listening to music with speakers in her ears. She was on the way to the store, just a short walk from her house. This young lady had to defend herself against an abduction! Can you imagine? Some sicko drove up next to her and offered her a ride. She declined, he offered again, she declined again, now catching on, and then he tried to drag her into his car to take her away. God only knows what foul things he had in mind. I shudder to think about it. I can't claim any credit for what happened next, as she had been learning Martial Arts for many years. Her instincts took over. She punched and punched and punched her way out. Thank God that she had training.

After this series of students had all told me crazy stories in a short time, my practice, study, and teaching of self-defense was reinvigorated. I have been blessed to study several different Martial Arts in great depth, with an amazing teacher and many great mentors. I set out to discover, using insight from everything that I had learned, what are the easiest, simplest, most effective strategies that could be used by everyone, regardless of skill, strength, size, and training. I studied how the body responds under stress, and what skills can you really use even in an adrenalized situation. My Martial Arts training had prepared me well, but it helped me to look at it with fresh eyes, and with new purpose. My concept and vision, so long in preparation, **Immediate Self Defense**, was born. Now I have taught my brainchild for many years, and heard from many more students their successful stories of Self Defense.

What are my Qualifications?

Everyone has something or several things that they can uniquely offer to the world. For me, it's my love of Martial Arts, and my passion for Self Defense. I am a Rotarian, and we believe in "Service Above Self." My way of serving the world is to share what I have learned, to help you stay safe for the benefit of your loved ones, your family, and your community. You are important. We need you. Please learn and take care of yourself so you can take care of others.

I have devoted my life to the study, practice, and especially the teaching of Martial Arts. In my lineage (line of succession of Martial Arts teachers), doing and teaching are considered separate skills. Sometimes the most gifted athletes do not make good coaches. Leadership skills are somewhat different than just learning to be excellent. You must learn how to inspire and motivate, to encourage and build up, and most of all, how to listen and adapt.

I have studied Martial Arts and Self Defense thoroughly, yes, but I have studied the teaching of Martial Arts and Self Defense probably even more. I have attended so many trainings and classes on Self Defense that I cannot count them all, and would struggle to remember all of the teachers' names. Always looking not so much for content or techniques, but for teaching strategies, studying what works and what doesn't and why. I strive to be the most effective teacher that I can be, especially to the people with whom I can have the greatest impact, people who are getting first exposure. Beginners. Or even people who don't even have an interest, until you inspire them, and awaken their interest and passions.

I love to give lectures, assemblies, and talk to people who have never seen or heard anything about Self Defense before. I love to give them their first exposure, or even if they have extensive experience, to give them a fresh way to look at what they know. Just the other day, a student in a workshop told me he had learned something from me that he had never seen before, and he had law enforcement and military special forces training! To me it was a normal thing, but he really valued it. A fresh perspective can be very useful.

I'll be the first to say that I am not the most gifted practitioner. I've suffered some serious injuries through my years of training that hamper my ability to perform at the level that I would like. However, I stay active in training, practice, and teaching, and always seek to improve. Most importantly, I want my students to be better than me!

Self Defense and Martial Arts Qualifications:
- Frequently lecture and teach classes on Self Defense in my community and at our local college
- Specialize in teaching the basics of Self Defense to beginners
- Creator of Immediate Self Defense
- The Self Defense instructor for NORBAR (North Bay Association of Realtors)
- Founder of the 501(c)3 non-profit Martial Arts Academy Bujutsu Gakuin Wushu Xueyuan
- Over 20 years of Martial Arts study
- Over 10 years teaching Martial Arts and Self Defense full time
- Sifu (Father Teacher) of Qi Xing Tang Lang Quan Fa (350 year old system of Kung Fu)
- Sensei (Teacher) of Okinawan Karate & Kobudo (Matsubayashi Ryu & Goju Ryu styles)
- Sensei (Teacher) of Japanese Swordsmanship (Iaido, Kenjutsu, Kendo, and Batto-Do)
- Instructor of Yang Style Tai Chi Chuan
- Senior Instructor, Chinese Athletic Arts Academy
- Certified 4th Degree Black Belt with USA Karate
- Kata Judge and Kumite Referee for USA Karate and Karate Referee Association
- Instructor for Karate Referee Association
- United States Olympic Committee Safesport Certified
- Shaolin Temple Educators Award from deceased Grandmaster

Ming Lum, Godfather of Kung Fu
* Chinese Martial Arts Judge for ICMAC, USA Wushu Kung Fu Federation, and TC Judges Union

Differences between Martial Arts & Self Defense

What is the difference between Martial Arts and Self Defense? Most people wouldn't recognize a difference. However, to me, they are VERY different. I'm sure my view is colored by my experience. Please allow my experience to be of benefit to you. The advantage of a focused self-defense course over a Martial Arts course is that in Martial Arts, you have many things to learn, and here you have only a few. With the course being a short duration, this is especially important. I have crystallized all my experience into a "least you need to know" kind of format to make it easy to absorb.

A Self Defense course is a terrific way to jump-start your Martial Arts journey. Kickboxing, Karate, Kung Fu, and other similar classes are a great way to stay in shape and work on impact training, vital for effective Self Defense. The most important part of your training is that you find the right place to do it. You want to be around a supportive group of friendly people. This makes it easy to do well, and makes you want to come to class! Consistency and a good attitude are the most important parts of training.

Traditional Martial Arts learned correctly are the epitome of Self Defense, and more. If you have studied Martial Arts for more than a couple years, then you should be familiar with all the things that we cover in this book, and many of the skills we would cover in our introductory Self Defense classes. Once we start getting in-depth, you may find skills that are unfamiliar to you, depending on your length, breadth, and depth of experience. Unfortunately, not all teachers of Martial Arts spent enough time as students themselves, or were not thoroughly trained how to teach, and what has happened over time is that many teachers and even systems have changed to become mostly mere exercise instead of effective self-defense.

Traditional Martial Arts offer many additional wonderful benefits, and a full range of techniques and strategies. You learn many different ways to use your body in traditional training, with the end goal of discovering what is natural and effective for you and your body type. Forms give you ways of practicing these effective techniques when you don't have a partner, and they also reinforce proper posture and body position, which makes all the difference in effective self-defense. The best part of forms is that you don't have a partner in your way, so you are able to practice your movements full out without a chance of injuring a training partner. Many people think traditional weapons training has no place in modern society, but in addition to being really fun and challenging, if you have to defend yourself, using a weapon can instantly increase your effectiveness. Each traditional weapon brings new awareness to your different joints and their use and position. When you have trained with several weapons, you will more easily understand difficult concepts such as range in much greater depth. These concepts are fundamental, but difficult to master.

To me, the difference between Self Defense and Martial Arts is primarily in scope: Self Defense is a much smaller and easier skillset, while Martial Arts is quite a large subject. There is a LOT to Martial Arts. Self Defense is something that EVERYONE should learn, regardless of how little time you may have to devote to it. A little bit of study goes a long way.

Self Defense is certainly PART of Martial Arts. You really aren't doing Martial Arts if you don't learn how to defend yourself, but Martial Arts is SO MUCH MORE. The next section of the book is going to explain the benefits of Martial Arts.

Benefits of Martial Arts

Martial Arts have many wonderful benefits to other forms of

physical training. There have recently been a lot of studies on the benefits of Martial Arts practice versus other types of exercise. If you do a quick google search, you can find many such examples for yourself. I'm not going to mention any specifics here, in case any links change or stop working, but you can find these studies easily enough.

Martial Arts training provides you with excellent physical training. You will get a structured warm-up that will get your body ready for exercise to prevent injury, some vigorous exercise which provides a mental and emotional release, you will connect your mind and body through choreographed movements with partners and without to program your nervous system for correct response in times of stress, and some cool-down and stretching exercises that will help prevent injury, relax you, and leave you feeling great.

Vigorous exercise helps regulate your stress responses, such as adrenaline and cortisol. When you experience stress but have no release such as exercise, it can lead to all sorts of negative effects such as: sleep disturbances, decreased bone density, decreased muscle mass, accumulation of abdominal fat, elevated blood pressure, and lower immune function.

It is natural for us to experience stress, and regular exercise can help us recover from the stress in a constructive way. Have you ever yelled at someone or treated them badly for no reason when they didn't deserve it? Likely you were under stress, and you would benefit from the release that exercise provides. I have found that impact training such as striking pads or heavy bags like we do in Martial Arts is especially satisfying for many people. When you get this release, your emotions are regulated, and you are able to be your best self for yourself and your loved ones. There is no way to completely eliminate stress, so it is important to learn how to bounce back and recover from stress.

Why don't people stay with exercise routines? Often it is because they don't have a peer group that they feel comfortable with that holds them accountable and misses them when they are not there. This is why I believe so strongly in a Martial Arts school atmosphere. There you should find a group of friendly, happy people, who support each other and are happy to see you. A proper atmosphere is very important, and it begins with the tone the teacher sets.

Besides the exercise benefits of Martial Arts, which are significant, there are many other benefits for you and your children. Martial Arts teach you to respect yourself, to respect others, to do your best, to never give up, and that Martial Arts are to be used for defense only. From this basis, these other benefits are possible: focus, self-confidence, social skills, discipline, problem solving, conflict resolution, breathing, concentration, dexterity, patience, listening, teamwork, posture, balance, memory, coordination, goals, endurance, humility, belief in yourself, good behavior at home and at school, and many more.

Many Martial Arts use a belt ranking system. The great thing about belt ranks is that they offer a series of increasing challenges. As you accomplish each belt, you are able to see, verify, and validate your progress. This is incredibly empowering. When you truly understand that the power of your own effort and work can lead to better and better results, you can go after your dreams and accomplish them.

The ultimate and original purpose of Martial Arts is to create leaders. Leaders are able to benefit society through their service in greater and greater ways. This is only possible when you have learned how powerful you can be as an example, through service, and that true power comes only through cooperation with and help of other people. If you are interested in these aspects of Martial Arts, I recommend www.leaderprinciples.com

Chapter 2
Why Immediate Self Defense

Stress Responses & Adrenaline

The body has certain predictable responses to stressful situations. If you think about it, I know you are familiar with them already, even if you've never had to defend yourself. Have you ever had to speak publicly? That is a huge stressor for a lot of people. Ever experienced road rage? How about been in a car accident? Or had a heated argument with someone?

If you've experienced anything like these, you have felt at least some of the effects I'm about to describe firsthand, so I know you can relate. Common effects of an adrenaline dump include: heart rate and respiratory changes, tunnel vision, loss of hearing, inability to take in and process new information, no fine motor skills, time dilation (moving fast, moving slow, inconsistent), increased speed and strength, loss of touch sensitivity including increased pain tolerance, unconscious movements or freezing, short term memory loss including non-formation of memory, no depth perception, and the list goes on. Not everyone has the same responses, and they can vary not only person to person but event to event. Adrenaline is said to affect people differently based on gender. From what I've seen and heard, I think this is generally true, though like anything, there are bound to be exceptions. Let's speak generally, then. Men and women tend to have similar amounts of adrenalin; however, their reactions to adrenaline are markedly different. Men get the adrenaline dump almost all at once and their bodies go crazy with ability, but they tend to experience more of the negative side-effects (such as tunneling, hearing loss, time dilation, and inability to process new information), and when adrenaline wears off, they are practically useless, physically spent, and unable to function well for a period of time. Think of a man's adrenaline dump as vertical. Incredibly strong, but short-lived benefits. With women, think of their adrenaline dump as horizontal instead. Adrenaline heightens their heart rate and changes their respiration, giving them advantages, but instead of causing extreme tunnel vision, hearing loss, and time dilation, many women are able to take in new information, listen and process words, and adjust to changing circumstances.

This is important to understand, because women might find it natural to talk to a man in a confrontation, to try to reason with him, or ask "why me?" but if the man is under the effect of adrenaline he may literally not be able to hear you, have an inability to take in new information, and even be left with no memory of what you said because the memories literally did not form.

It has been explained to me this way: that our creator made men to fight the monsters by becoming the monster, while making women able to take the children and flee and even protect them until it is safe to return. I hope you can pardon me for mentioning this rather sexist and old-fashioned way of looking at the world, but I believe the visual it creates rather accurately describes how adrenaline affects our genders.

With time and exposure to stresses, the body gradually acclimatizes, so people who work in extremely stressful environments become accustomed to them and are able to function at a higher level when in their normal work environment. (Think 911 operators, EMTs, Paramedics, Firemen, Law Enforcement, Military Personnel, etc.)

Less to Remember – Easy Works

For those of you who teach Martial Arts, please remember that if a person has not trained extensively, and undergone adrenalized

14

training, complicated and detailed techniques that rely on fine motor skills will simply not be available to them, and will instead cause them to freeze and fixate on why it is not working. Fight and flight are both great responses, but freeze is a common response that we have to do specific training to get past, and you don't want to trigger it unnecessarily.

The reason Martial Arts get so complicated is that, yes, there are absolutely ideal ways of responding to any possible attack. Martial Arts usually teach you 3-5 ways to respond to anything, and with practice, you discover what you like, and improve your weak areas. Then in higher level training, you practice under stress and those skills become usable. All of the top teachers that I have worked with have understood this and made it part of their high level, closed door, or private training for their most elite students.

But without this extensive amount of experience, similar to what a high level black belt, bodyguard or law enforcement officer would love to have, having too many options and things to remember cause a civilian or casual Self Defense student to freeze, hesitate, doubt themselves, and get caught in a loop of failure (the mind sometimes can't process why something isn't working and will repeat).

If you need to defend yourself, do you want to have to comb through your memory to find the appropriate best response? If you've read an earlier part of this book where we talk about adrenaline dump and stress response, you will realize that even if you want to, unless you have an incredible amount of experience, you cannot. The part of your brain that allows you to think of the best response won't be available to you, and you won't have time to figure it out before it is all over (confrontations happen incredibly quickly and are resolved just as fast). Trying to sift through hundreds of possible responses that way will just cause you to freeze, and do nothing in response to the attack, which will be harmful if not fatal.

Immediate Self Defense is designed to be the very easiest responses that you could have. There are less decisions to make, less possible choices, only a few things to remember, and they are designed that if you make a mistake you just keep going and it will work. You do not have to try and fail and try something else and go in a loop. Our concepts are simple, and work with your body's natural responses. The best part is, Immediate Self Defense is designed to take all possible advantage of your body's natural leverages, so even if you are small, weak, or infirmed, you are a formidable opponent. (I have had the pleasure to work with a few very short but incredibly formidable teachers, most notably Hanshi Nakamoto Masahiro who is under 5' tall, but incredibly strong, and the now deceased Professor Imi Okazaki-Mullins, who was very small and frail the last time I worked with her, but she could still throw me across a room, seemingly without effort. This was quite surprising to me because I am a large 6' tall man!)

In the hands-on classes, we introduce concepts by showing you why and how they work exactly, and make sure you get to really feel them. We work them in a variety of variations and from different angles, so you get a complete picture of them. I think it is important to explore why other things do NOT work so your body gets a visceral memory of failure from bad strategies and success from proper ones. Each Immediate Self Defense concept is really easy to use, easy to understand, and works seemingly like magic. For those who do more in-depth training like we offer at our weekend intensives, we can help you feel an adrenalized state safely, and let you work through your body's responses. This high level training is truly invaluable. Once you have trained your responses enough in an adrenalized state, you know how you will react, and know that you are trained and safe.

Usually, training like this is only available to the select few. I make it available to the general public much more quickly, because I believe it can make the difference between life and death. If you are interested, please contact me. There is a process we have to work through, and we have to get to know and trust each other so that it is safe. We do these trainings at intensive weekends and in private instruction, not in general classes.

Body Mechanics

The fundamentals of human body mechanics are pretty well understood these days. As a species, we are very adept at using our bodies in all kinds of ways. Even without any training, most people can do quite a bit with their bodies. However, with hands on training, you can learn to use the maximum mechanical advantage in everything you do.

In my introductory workshops, I make it a point to explore by demonstration and hands-on testing, how some of the fundamentals of body mechanics really work. People find that portion very eye opening, and it is often one of their favorite parts. I've had a huge number of very highly coordinated people, dancers and gymnasts and athletes of all kinds take my class. The more they know about their bodies, the more they like the class. The fact is, in Martial Arts, we are specialists in not only how to use our bodies, but how to use our bodies when we clash with other forces, another body, or multiple other bodies. We learn to use our bodies under pressure, and that is similar yet different from many other kinds of athletics.

Just last month, I saw a former student, who had taken an introductory class a couple years ago. She said that she had loved it so much and had gotten so much out of it. She said that she had not had to defend herself or anything like that, and she loved all the awareness exercises, but what had made a huge difference in her life was understanding body mechanics. She told me that she had suffered back pain most of her life, and by applying the principles she learned in my class, she was moving so much differently that her back pain was gone. Those are what we call atypical results. Awesome for sure, but I'm not saying you should expect that. Still, when you move your body in an ideal way, everything is easier.

When teaching body mechanics for Self Defense, I start with how force affects posture and structure. I find that is the easiest way to get people who are just starting out to really get the feel of how their posture and structure make a difference. Hands-on learning in person is the only way to experience this, and it has to be from a teacher who really understands well.

We work on movement and pressure quite a bit. In real life, untrained people fall down all the time, and then they really get in trouble. Sure, on the TV you might see two people wrestling around on the ground and it might go either way, but do you realize that in real life it's almost never one on one? Because you are frequently outnumbered, doing ground techniques is a last resort. And everything you think you know about groundfighting changes when you also have to defend against someone standing up as well as someone wrestling with you. All of that is important to learn, but we start with something more fundamental: learn to move your feet and respond to pressure, and try at all costs to avoid going to the ground. It works well. After learning these principles, I have never been taken to the ground unless I wanted to go there. Too many people today focus on the groundfighting part without focusing on body movement. Also, what you see on TV has rules. Don't do that in real Self Defense. If you are being assaulted, don't wrestle. If a person is leaning over, their leverages are all different, so we work on how to exploit that to our advantage. Self Defense isn't a sport. You must be willing to be as brutal as necessary, using only the techniques that are so effective they are unsafe for sporting competition, to ensure you are safe.

The key principle we apply in all our concepts is this – use the entire mass of your body on a tiny area of the criminal's body. This is how I can teach children to defend themselves successfully against an adult. Never fight force with force. Move, and use everything you've got at the weakest spots, and you can break free from any grip, and make any situation better.

We learn their anatomical weak spots for striking and leverage, and our concepts exploit those only. No low percentage techniques. Only what works immediately.

No Memorization

If you are studying Self Defense with me, there is almost nothing to memorize. There are some fundamental concepts that have to be felt, experienced, and practiced quite a bit. But we do away completely with a decision tree of what is appropriate for what. If you teach Martial Arts, you frequently get asked the question, "But what if I do this instead?" There is always a counter to every counter, and that discussion is endless. The reason it happens is because in Martial Arts, we make things very complicated. We teach a minimum of 3-5 strategies for every possible scenario, and that is just step one of the engagement. Then once they resist this way there is this variation, and if they resist this other way there is this other variation. I actually enjoy this training too, but it is very cerebral. Things simply don't work that way when you apply real speed and force. It can be a useful tool to teach you how your body and theirs can work, but it's nothing like real life. You don't get to use that part of your brain unless you have hundreds of hours of real life experience in confrontations. In the old days of Martial Arts, they were only practiced by people who used them for real every day.

That level of skill is quite uncommon today. In higher level training today, we are more like Bruce Lee. He didn't invent this concept, but he famously said words to the effect that you don't want to accumulate more each day, you want to get rid of more each day. What we mean by this in Martial Arts is that you may have learned 3-5 or 10 ways to do something in order to get a certain rank. Great! Now pick one, and do it 10,000 times so you can really use it.

If you are physically assaulted, it happens very quickly, and there is simply no time to run through a bunch of possible ideas and make choices. Another consideration is visual too – you very well may not be able to see exactly how you are being assaulted! Imagine the problem of having only practiced with perfect vision and with time to be able to figure out what to do, and working slowly. That is great practice for beginners or to introduce new concepts, but you must get past it in real practice or you will never be truly effective in real life.

If you have to stop and think, and use what I call a decision tree where you think of what move provokes what response, you are in big trouble. This takes too much time, and in the panicked mode that you will find yourself in should you need to defend yourself, you will not be able to do it. Worse yet, it may take you out of Fight or Flight, and right into Freeze, the dangerous response that we need to avoid at all costs.

Because there is nothing to memorize, every response happens naturally and automatically. My students frequently comment that the techniques seem almost to be magic, and that once you get used to them, it seems impossible not to do them. They are natural by design, taking advantage of the instincts that are native to our human bodies, which we will discuss in the next section.

So Immediate Self Defense is very different than the Self Defense portions of many Martial Arts because they are greatly simplified. I have learned that without extensive training, people simply cannot apply very many moves, and cannot remember what to do. That's why my program is designed with no memorization, and only natural, easy movements.

Instinctual

Everything I teach is instinctual. What this means is it takes advantage of the automatic responses that your body has to stress, pressure, and assault. There are certain things that all human bodies are hardwired to do. It is extremely difficult to change these responses, and that level of training is not something that is attained by most people, because it must be done under pressure, thousands upon thousands of times.

Instead, Immediate Self Defense is based on these autonomic responses that your body will have, which makes them automatic, instinctual, rapid, and impossible to get wrong. Our concepts are not based on fine motor skill which deteriorates under high blood pressure (your blood pressure goes through the roof in a real situation) and adrenaline. Instead, what I teach is based on the absolutely most gross motor movement possible by design – those motions which you can do no matter what. Frankly, this is the only way to be effective unless you have logged thousands of hours of practice under pressure.

Because Immediate Self Defense works with both what is hardwired into your nervous system as autonomic (automatic, without thought), responses, and with gross motor movement (biggest muscles, least degree of complication), the concepts seemingly work like magic. It is exceedingly difficult if not impossible to resist techniques applied in this way.

We take it a couple steps further, however, to make sure that it works against people of all sizes. Children are able to effectively use these concepts against adults who might be trying to abduct them because of these next key points.

We make sure we put all of our mass in motion to accomplish our result. It's simple, really. We get more bang for the buck if we are using our whole body then if we are ever just using our limbs. We practice moving and moving and moving and responding to pressure. This helps us break down the freeze response so that it is less likely, and more easy to recover from if you find that it IS your natural response (like so many people today find). Don't worry if that's you.

With a little practice, we can significantly alter that result. The freeze response is mostly a sign of too much cerebral activity, not enough physicality. I seldom find a person who has several years of training in athletics who has a freeze response. By adding just a little bit of physicality into your daily life, you can virtually eliminate the freeze response in a short time.

As we practice moving, we are conscious to stay off the ground however possible. Most real life situations are not one on one, so this means that if you are on the ground, you likely have at least one assailant standing over you while you wrestle with another. This is a deadly place to be. Movement is always preferable. So in our beginning classes we work on all the movements that can keep you off the ground and mobile, taking any chance to get away. We learn the leverages and how they work so that you cannot be easily controlled, and you have a better chance to slip away and escape. In our intensive weekends, we practice transitioning from standing to the ground and back to standing with single and multiple opponents, working on stepping and movement to slip and evade. These concepts take time to become second nature, and intensive training is the best way to learn them. You must feel them fully.

One last note on instinct. It is important how you practice. There is a famous true story of a police officer who practiced a gun disarm technique thousands upon thousands of times. Each time, he would hand the gun back to his partner right away so they could practice again. Then one day he had to use the technique in real life. A criminal drew a gun, and he took it away. However, because of his poor training method and not understanding how the nervous system gets programmed, he automatically HANDED THE GUN RIGHT BACK TO THE CRIMINAL!

In traditional Martial Arts, because their lessons were learned by hard won experience, we are taught after a disarm to clear the area, and to remove ourselves from the situation. We practice with what the Japanese call Zanshin, a lingering feeling, a remaining mind, an active readiness, realizing that the confrontation is not over until it is over.

Avoidance before Engagement

A lot of people who teach Self Defense seem to only be interested in the physical aspects of it, and frankly, they do it all wrong, making it more complicated than it should be, and less effective. They emphasize the wrong points.

Truthfully, the most important thing you could learn that would help you the most is avoidance of the problem in the first place. If you can learn avoidance before engagement, you are really ahead of the game. Engaging should be the last resort. Avoidance has failed. That's why we learn that Martial Arts are for defense only. One of our oldest manuals of Martial Arts and strategy, SunZi's Art of War, says that to win 100 victories in 100 battles is not the highest skill, but to win WITHOUT fighting is the highest skill. If you successfully avoid a confrontation, if you avoid before engage, you have won.

For some people, because of Ego, they are not able to see the benefit of winning without fighting. The immature Ego mind would rather have you walk across a dark park with poor visibility because you feel that it ought to be safe, rather than facing the reality that it exposes you to undue risk, and you could simply walk around in the streetlights. You don't have to take every invitation to get in a fight. There is often an opportunity to avoid things before they start. If someone is mouthing off to you and you mouth off back and it escalates, it will become a fight. You are both at fault. The immature ego mind will not allow you a way out. If you feel wronged or slighted in some way, you will want to fight back. If they use words to egg you on or make you feel small, your ego will force you to take regrettable action. Remember this: If you wrestle with a pig, you both get dirty, and the pig enjoys it. If you are not actively being attacked, there is time to do something else to try to avoid the confrontation. Get outta there. Swallow your pride. It is worth it. I wish you could see it as clearly as I do, you would not make that mistake. If you were mature enough to look at the real cost, you would make a better decision for yourself.

If you do, in fact, defend yourself, and it was a situation that you could have avoided, there are a lot of crazy thoughts that will occur to you. You will feel powerful that you defended yourself. You will feel weak and foolish that you got into the situation. You will feel great that you know you are capable. You will feel foolish that you did not walk away. These days, you will probably end up both of you filing a complaint against each other, possibly going to jail. Depending on how each of you was injured, etc, and how good your lawyers are, you will end up paying a SIGNIFICANT amount of time and money, and quite possibly giving up a portion of your life or your potential (jail time and/or a record that will follow you for life). If your assailant is a criminal, he will know the system better than you, and know just what to say, and he will have nothing to lose. It will be his word against yours.

For many of those reasons, running is starting to look like a much better option than before, isn't it? I hope so. The old Chinese expression is that if you are patient in one moment of anger, you will avoid 100 days of sorrow.

Some people have to learn the hard way. I hope that if you are reading this book, you will take the long view on your life, and realize the value of avoidance before engagement. If you think only in terms of earning potential, if because of felonies you can only earn half (many jobs will not allow felons), will that allow you to provide for yourself and your family? A criminal felon has nothing to lose, while you have everything to lose.

Chapter 3
Understanding the Criminal Mindset

Why Me?

It is perfectly normal to have this thought if you are attacked: "Why Me?" However, the truth is, at that moment, it doesn't matter. If you are being attacked, you need to focus on getting out of there and getting safe. You need to push the "why me" and all distracting thoughts from your mind, because you are busy! Some people call it "condition black" or "code black." Give it any name you want, but if you are under attack, it's time to let your deep nature take over. The oldest parts of your brain regulate things like breathing and heart rate. Let the reaction come; you can't stop it anyway. Resistance is futile. Then the next part of your brain will signal the adrenaline dump. You may feel it coming on. This is extremely good. This is how your body was designed to respond to stress to give you the best chance of survival. Don't try to think of what to do. This will only delay you. Just let your body do what is natural. Fight back, and don't stop fighting back until you are able to break away and get safe.

We modern humans have life very easy compared to our predecessors, from whom we inherited our brains and their functioning. The majority of us will never see war, or real life and death struggle in person, and only a percentage of us will see true violence up close and personal (and hopefully, since you are reading this book, you will learn how to avoid it so you never have to see it!).

I want to leave you a thought here. Every one of us who lives in a modern, industrialized nation who does not have to struggle each day for our survival is in a significantly different position than our predecessors. However, if you have ever paid any attention to the news, things can flip in an instant. Places that had been peaceful and safe can almost instantly be turned around to become life or death because of natural disasters, to use one example. Think of the frequency of looting that breaks out whenever there is the slightest provocation. If you are paying attention, you realize that we are not so far removed from violence. It is, in fact, in our nature. I didn't write that to scare you, but I never want you to take for granted the importance of manners.

Manners did not evolve from polite societies. They evolved from successful warrior traditions who wished for peace. The best warriors could certainly fight, but they preferred peace. Peace allows everyone to thrive, and for all sorts of things to exist that cannot exist in war, such as trade. True warriors have always sought to keep the peace, so you should learn manners. If you acted with poor manners in times past, there could be dire consequences. Even today, try saying the wrong thing to a gang member and see what happens to you! I did that once, and ended up with my car broken into by his gang friends, but that story is in another chapter. The importance of treating people well cannot be overstated. You will make mistakes, but apologize sincerely, and treat them well, and it is better than if you don't.

Think of your emotions when someone treats you poorly, or you feel disrespected, slighted, ignored, marginalized, etc. The bad feelings you get can fester, and become worse than they should be. Pretty soon you don't even know what caused the original bad feelings, you just know you don't like someone. The event may even have been a simple misunderstanding, or may look completely different from the other person's point of view. This is the root of many of our problems in society.

Treat people well. You will save yourself a lot of problems, hassle, and inconvenience. When you treat people well and give them a chance to be important, they will like you and you have made an ally and a friend. Hold your temper in one moment of anger, or you may cause a lifetime of regret.

Crimes of Opportunity

90% of crimes are crimes of opportunity. This means that the criminal is not looking for you specifically, they are just looking for an easy target. There are a lot of ways that you can show yourself to be an easy target, and there are also ways that you can demonstrate that you are a hard target, and they should take their business elsewhere. It's pretty straightforward. If you do not leave the opportunity, the criminal will choose someone else.

I'm going to start with a classic example I've heard teachers talk about more times than I can count. I call this example "the shopper." In this example, you are Christmas shopping, and have far too many bags in your hands. You carry everything to your car, and then fumble around for your keys. All of this has provided a LOT of opportunity for a criminal.

A less extreme example of the same thing could be if you are on the phone on your way to your car, then arriving at your car you fumble in your purse or pockets for your keys. Again, this provides a lot of potential exposure to a criminal.

Not as many people talk all the time on the phone; now more often, we are texting. This is even worse for awareness in many ways, as you are looking down at your phone, and have less possibility of looking around and identifying danger as you go.

You might be distracted, mentally preoccupied and lost in thought. If you are out and about, that also puts you at greater risk, because it makes you an easy target. If you are not paying attention, you are an easy target for a criminal.

If you have visible cash, expensive jewelry or electronic devices, you are a target to a criminal on the lookout for a quick score. (Two of my students have had their electronic devices stolen right out of their hands when they were in public places by a person who rapidly disappeared into the crowd, and they did not even get a decent look at them.)

So far, our examples have all been if you are alone. If you are alone, you are a more accessible target for a single criminal. However, even if you are with someone else, you can still be an attractive target. If you are arguing, then you are clearly not paying attention and are heavily distracted. Save arguing for private time, not public time when you could have criminal exposure. I know many of these suggestions seem highly unusual, but I hope you can see their value.

I hate to say it, but women are highly likely to need to defend themselves at some point in their lives. I generally don't quote statistics because they are a funny thing. You can find statistics that prove and disprove almost any point. However, from all my research, it seems that over 100% of women are the victims of violent crimes. This number, though, does not mean all women suffer violent crimes, because some women are victims of violent crimes several times. It does, however, clearly show the need for women to learn Self Defense. It's bad enough that women desperately need to defend themselves. However, there is another group that is assaulted even more than women.

The visibly infirm (meaning appearing weak) through age, visible injury, or illness are highly likely to be assaulted by criminals, because it is thought that they won't have the strength to defend themselves. Just like criminals frequently try to defraud the elderly, some scumbags outright attack them. These same criminals choose people who are on crutches or whose arms are in a sling etc. to attack. Makes me so angry I almost want to pull out an old set of crutches, put my arm in a sling, and go out with money hanging out of my pockets.

Hmm... on second thought, I guess I'm a little too smart to do that without police backup. Hey, why don't they do that? I guess it would be entrapment. Too bad. I wonder if the criminals would fall for it. I'll let you know next week. Just kidding. I think. Maybe.

How to be a Hard Target

If you are a hard target, that means that the criminal does not want to choose you to deal with. By their very nature, criminals are looking for an easy target, one that provides little challenge and offers great reward. If they wanted to work hard, they'd go get a job. It is because of this inherent laziness that you have a great advantage if you are willing and able to become a hard target. They will choose someone else! It's not YOU they're targeting, it's an exploitable opportunity.

To become a hard target, here are habits you want to cultivate: assertiveness, stand tall, head up, eye contact, voice loud and strong, wallet in front pocket or purse held under the arm instead of dangling by the straps, comfortable clothes and shoes that allow easy movement.

Pretend for a moment that you are a criminal. I know, I know, it's uncomfortable, but bear with me. Now, there are two ladies walking down the street. Both look professional, and are well dressed. One has on a tight dress that might restrict her movement, high heels, and is holding her purse by a single strap. The other has on a business suit, sensible shoes, and has her arm through the strap of her purse and under her arm. If you are a criminal, which one would you pick to take their purse? Probably most of you picked the one in heels who might have a harder time running after you, who was barely holding onto her purse. If you picked the other lady, congratulations! You would make a terrible criminal, better keep your day job. Now that example was obvious, right? But there are plenty of people who go around like the first lady in our example.

Do you know that many criminals perform little tests for target selection? It goes like this. They look around, and find someone who seems introverted. Someone who has their head down, and when they look at their eyes, the person looks down and hunches their shoulders. If that's you, that's a problem, because you just indicated submissiveness in a big way to the human predator. Criminals who have been at it very long know that many people simply won't report crimes. It is too difficult to deal with, too much hassle, and they don't have enough self-esteem to realize that they are worth it and don't deserve this kind of trouble! The worst thing is, the people who act submissive like this the most are usually people who have a history of abuse and/or violence. They may have been victims of violent crime before, and it may not even be worth it to them to report. The system is especially ineffective at punishing criminals if there's any way to let them go, and sometimes victims themselves end up feeling victimized by the system. If you have been abused, you likely either continue to be abused, or frequently become an abuser yourself. It's a horrible cycle of life. We model the behaviors we see; monkey see, monkey do.

The same if a criminal tries to talk to you and you look away because you are uncomfortable and mumble something or other. You send them a clear signal that you are wishy-washy, and a good target for them. If instead you get a bad vibe when they get much too close and you say "leave me alone" or "back off" in a loud, clear voice, you show them that you are a tough cookie, and they will choose another target instead. A criminal may act like it was all a misunderstanding and no big deal, but don't be fooled, and don't doubt yourself. Leave the area and check your purse/wallet. You have that sixth sense for a reason. It is quite real and useful.

If you are the victim of a crime, and you can identify the criminal, please report it and see it through. Often criminals face much reduced consequences simply because there isn't enough in their background to show a pattern of violent or criminal behavior. It all starts with a victim being strong enough to stand up to the criminal and see it through for the good of everyone. Yes it is an inconvenience. Yes it takes time. Yes it can be very hard to do as a victim when you are already mentally and emotionally overloaded. Yes I think it's worth it.

One Crime Leads to Another

I'll tell you now a little story. It seems like a joke, but there's no punch line. Once upon a time I worked as a janitor overnight at a hotel. This was more than twenty years ago now. I was new to the area and going to school in the morning, and this job gave me just the schedule I needed. There was a young kid who worked with me who, I found out, was in a gang. I was pretty new to Northern California, and I had never met a person in a gang from up here. Frankly I didn't think there really were gangs here. In some places there are quite serious gangs, but as far as I had seen, this area was really relaxed, and there was no serious gang activity anywhere around.

I had the bad idea of giving him a hard time about being part of a gang, telling him that his gang was probably just a bunch of punk kids and that if he continued to be part of it, he would turn out to be a loser. Who was I to say all that? Whether I was right or wrong, I should have considered my audience, and kept my opinion to myself. He got upset, and I blew him off. After that, he started treating me much better, and for some reason, I didn't take it as the warning sign that I should have. Instead, he put me at ease and I let my guard down even further. A couple days went by, and then he said to me, "Hey man, you got that older blue car, right?" I didn't connect the dots and said "Yeah, the one over in this spot" and plainly described the location of my car. Honestly, sometimes I think part of why I'm equipped to write this book is because I've made every stupid mistake a person could make. Don't share unsolicited opinions about other people's lives and choices. Ever. And consider carefully if your opinion, even if they ask for it, would benefit them or just cause you and them both a bunch of grief.

Another couple days went by, and that coworker had quit suddenly and with no explanation. Then one morning I went to my car to quickly drive to school like always. The door was unlocked. I didn't notice. I quickly sat down (did I sit on something?) Oh well, in a hurry, I started the car. I would figure it out as I drove. Somehow I then noticed that it was really cold in the car (the passenger window had been broken and the entire contents of my car had been thrown around and dug through). I had a test that morning, so I thought for a second that I would just deal with it later. But as I started to quickly go through my stuff, and get it organized for school, I realized that my registration was missing. That somehow woke me up. I went back inside, and had human resources call police. When the police came, they took a report, explained that there had been a series of similar incidents around town. What they said next really hit home. I was asked if my registration was missing. It was. They ran my plates and got my registration, and sent a car to my house. My house was fine. Phew! I was ok. Unfortunately, I had just recently moved, and the registration with my new address had not come yet. The thieves had gotten the old address off the old registration. I got a call later that day that the thieves had gone and burglarized that old address. The police were quite disappointed that neither they nor I had connected the dots and thought of that other older address. However, they believed me that I was very distracted and hadn't even thought of it.

I was quite on edge the next few days. I thought that the gang would realize that it hadn't been my house that they burglarized, and that they would come back and get me after work some morning. It was causing me a lot of stress, and I wasn't sleeping well. I decided for peace of mind that I would quit that job. People who have any kind of trauma, no matter how minor like mine was, might react in quite irrational and over the top ways like I did.

Remember that I was trying to leave that morning in a hurry to get to school? My teacher for the class I was rushing off to, funny enough, didn't believe me, and said I faked the police report (what must he have seen to believe that?). He wouldn't let me make up the test and gave me an F, which plummeted my decent grade. I started trying to contest it with the college, but gave up amidst the bureaucracy of the whole situation and dropped the class. This caused a new problem, in that by dropping the class late, I was now going to get a W (withdraw) on my record, which would cause me other problems. I learned a valuable lesson, though, and it has helped me to have compassion for people in many circumstances. When people react to stressful events, they often cause themselves no end of additional problems and truly deserve compassionate help that will get them through. If you are mentally and emotionally dealing with a lot, you do not have the energy to do much. Even if it is relatively minor and "all in my head" like my situation was. Only one tiny thing had happened, but in my mind, it could have exploded and become much worse. Imagine how much worse it is for a victim of a serious violent crime like rape. If you know someone dealing with something like that, please give them all the support that you can.

Specifically Targeted by a Criminal

Okay, so if crimes of opportunity are 90% of crimes, what about the other 10%? This is the percentage that requires much better preparation and training to deal with. If you cannot avoid the issue, it can even require physical skills. Now if you are adept at removing every opportunity from a criminal, you may be able to prevent them having the opportunity to target you. Realistically, however, if a criminal has it out to get a certain person, and they keep their intentions hidden so you can't figure it out so you can avoid it, they will catch you by surprise. If they are patient and prepared, they will wait for the opportunity, and they will attack you.

Thank goodness most criminals are impatient, and are looking for an easy target, because the criminal who targets you personally and gives you no warning will really catch you by surprise. You would have no reason to be vigilant, and you would end up leaving some opportunity that they could exploit. It is inevitable.

It is in this situation that physical skills are an absolute necessity. In addition to physical skills, if your intuition is astute, you have a big advantage. Besides physical skills and intuition, if you have trained your mindset as we discuss in the next chapter, you will also have a distinct advantage. Your awareness will be your biggest asset. If you can see or feel something coming before it happens, and many of you can and do, then you can take action and get out of there. If you know where the exits are, you can run for them. Remember that if you can run, you should run. Running works the absolute best. If you can't run you should fight, and the moment you create the opportunity to run, you should run.

When you get away, you MUST report the assault to the police. Too many people manage to get away and get safe, but don't take action to report it. This is a real problem, because without those reports, the criminal doesn't have as much of a record, and cannot be seen as the threat they are.

Look, I hate to sound 'weird,' but I'm willing to do that to help you be safe. If you are in a situation and it feels uncomfortable, I want you to leave. Just leave first, and work out later if that was necessary or not. Your safety is really important. You are important. You have a lot to offer your family, your friends, and your community. We need you. You need to take care of yourself and get yourself out of harm's way.

Your 'sixth sense' or intuition is not a joke. We have great sensory organs: hearing, smell, taste, sight, and touch. However, the so-called sixth sense, intuition, is our most powerful. We may not totally understand it in scientific terms yet, but we all use it. This is the sense that gives us a feeling of impending doom right before something bad happens. This is the sense that makes us hesitate when we are about to do something and it just doesn't feel right. Call it whatever you like, but learn to listen to its messages, and pay attention to its commands. If you will train it, you will find it quite useful.

After training my intuition, more than once I have been in a crowded place and gotten a strange feeling. I looked around until I could figure out why. A man who I believe was a criminal seemed to be looking for a target. When I identified that it was him and I started looking hard at him and mentally going through the points for a physical description for police, he took off running. Now why would someone do that? And more than once? Different people, different places, same feeling. That's too weird, don't you think? To me it's not weird at all, and I can only explain it by saying, "it's intuition."

Perhaps, you, like me, are not convinced that time is entirely linear and proceeding only from beginning to end. If that's the case, perhaps we are picking up on flashes of possible futures that haven't reached full probability or permanence yet. Quantum theory is quite complicated, but it seems that Schrödinger's cat may exist simultaneously in more than one state until acted on by an outside force, the observer. "There are more things in heaven and earth, Horatio, than are dreamt of in your philosophy." Sorry to get weird again. Whatever the reason and however you explain it, what matters to me is the practical. You should invest time in listening to your intuition and training it, because it is a useful tool, and can keep you safe.

Known Persons

Did you know that some huge percentage (sources vary), of attackers are people that are known to the victims? How could it be? Well, you could be assaulted by someone that you know VERY well, like a spouse or immediate family member. It could also be an extended family member that assaults you because of some slight, real or imagined. Things also change dramatically with alcohol and drug use. If people are under the influence, boundaries are down, behaviors are risky, and there is greater likelihood of violent escalation. It's extremely risky to try to defend yourself by being gentle, thinking "it's only _____." While it may make sense to think this way when seen from the outside, when you are actually defending yourself, these vital moments can make the difference between life and death. Those thoughts that you shouldn't take it seriously, or they are drunk, or you both are, etc, those are very risky. Reality is that things happen quickly, and can go to hell in a handbasket far more quickly than you might realize. Once bad, they tend to get worse, not better.

There are also people who appear normal in most any way, except they have some form of mental illness. For those people, they may not form normal relationship bonds, and may instead, bond inappropriately to people that are little known to them (casual acquaintance, or even less, like someone you have run into a couple times at a coffee shop). Think of this as a dangerous twist on someone who has a big crush on a celebrity or famous athlete. If you don't know them well, there is not a real relationship, because it is just one-sided. However, it is entirely possible to build up fantasies of all different kinds with events that are minor or almost imagined (our hands touched when we both reached for the coffee). Don't get too caught up thinking about these kinds of things. There's no way to control what goes on in other people's heads. Most of us have a hard enough time controlling what goes on in our OWN heads.

The important thing to know for Self Defense in this case, is that it doesn't matter who is assaulting you. If you are under attack, you have the right to defend yourself. (Now, I'm no lawyer, so this is not legal advice, ok? Use your common sense and act appropriately for your jurisdiction/region/etc.) If you spend time considering their relationship to you (but it's just my uncle Bob), you are in big trouble. Do you realize how quickly things can get super serious and then resolve one way or the other? You don't have time for all those doubts.

If you are actually under attack, you need to fight back, hard, and find the opportunity to run away. That's right. You read that right. Do not stay and fight. I don't care how well trained you are, you get out of there. If you stay around, they may come after you. Most any situation these days is not one on one. And when you deal with two or more people, you cannot afford to stick around and try to talk to them to get them to stop (if you read the part about adrenaline, you understand that talking physiologically cannot work). Get away and call 9-1-1 (or whatever your emergency services number is). File a police report. It's a bit of a hassle (not too bad), but it's worth it. Do it for someone who doesn't get away. Help build a record on a criminal so the police and the lawyers can do what they need to do.

What happens all too often is that a person who is truly a repeat offender does not get a record, or does not have the record that they SHOULD have, because people did not report things like they should and could have. I've heard that people are "not surprised" that so and so did something bad because they were known for such and so, and then you hear about 5 stories of the past. Why did no one report? Seemingly minor things can quickly lead to far far greater things. It's a difficult job for law enforcement to connect the dots and prosecution to build cases; let's not make it harder for them.

Chapter 4
Self Defense Mindset

Rule #1 - Fight back and never give up

I cannot emphasize enough how important it is to fight back. In a situation where you need to defend yourself, there are a lot of factors. The psychology of the criminal is important to understand. Let's discuss this now. It is totally inappropriate to think about the psychology when you are under attack, there is no time. However, now, while we are safe, is the time to learn how things work so you can apply those lessons should you ever need them.

Looking at the basics of predator and prey psychology, you can begin to understand a criminal mindset during a confrontation. If you don't fight back, that demonstrates to the criminal that he picked a good target; you will be easy prey. He will become more aggressive and exhibit other dominant traits. He will tend to be worse even than he would have been because he will feel he can get away with it and you will do nothing.

Now it's totally different if you fight back. Fighting back begins with your posture, back erect and strong, your voice, loud, strong, and resistant ("back off" and "leave me alone") work well. Fighting back continues with all forms of physical resistance. Remember that a criminal wants an easy target who will not make noise and draw attention, and who will not fight back. Most of my students' success stories in Self Defense have to do with how they were not an easy target, and the criminal left them alone almost before it began. That's very effective Self Defense. Sometimes in those situations, you aren't even sure if it really WAS Self Defense, but let me tell you, if you de-escalated or avoided something before it really got going, you did a great job. It's good Self Defense.

If you haven't thought things through, or don't have much experience in real life, you might think that you should not offer much resistance, and look for a good opportunity to resist later on when the criminal is off guard. Sometimes we read, hear, or see things in media that give us the idea that it is good strategy to play along to get the criminal's guard down. The reality, however, is that there will never be a better time to resist than the moment of the initial assault. You simply cannot allow them to establish control if it is in any way in your power to prevent it. You have no way of knowing what they may do once they get control. They may have ties to bind you, gags so you can't make noise, or a way of making you pass out, so you will be compliant while they take you somewhere else. You simply can't afford to wait to resist. You must fight back.

If you are fighting back, you must keep up the resistance. You should be trying to find the opportunity to get away, because distance is your friend. At no time should you stop fighting. You must fight and you must never give up. As soon as you give up the fight, you have lost. At that moment, they will get control of you and you will be in a bad spot. Fortunately, your body is designed to help you to fight and to never give up. Adrenaline and its effects on the body allow you to do what is necessary. And remember that you are fighting for your life, while the criminal is not. He is only fighting for his dinner, so to speak.

Remember that your ultimate goal is very different than his. You are fighting to get away and get safe. All you need is one moment when he is not at his best, and you can achieve this. If he has any hesitation or doubt, you will achieve this. If he is unbalanced for even the briefest of moments, you will achieve this. It is really not as difficult as you might imagine.

Once you have broken free, you will be running for your life. We will address this in the next section. For now, what you need to know is that your goal is not to "take a criminal down" or to "take him out." Unless it is a single criminal, you have a lot of training, and you are prepared to trade your life for theirs, it is my advice to run if you are able. In a later chapter on defense of your family, we will address what to do if you are not "mobile," not able to get away, and must stop a criminal in their tracks. However, if you are a civilian and not law enforcement, in many areas, it is not even legal for you to restrain a criminal, so this should not be part of your thought process, unless it must be.

Running, the Best Option

Without question, the best option is running. Distance is your friend in self-defense, like no other. Handheld weapons of all types (like sticks and knives) cannot reach you and become ineffective with enough distance. Even firearms are less effective with more distance.

Even with training, it is risky to fight with your bare hands against someone armed. If you are facing a stick, club, baton, baseball bat, or anything blunt, you will be hit. Moving out of range completely is a great option if you can run away. However, with sufficient training, you can understand that moving away but not out of range can make the impact more. If you make the decision to disarm, you will learn which parts of your anatomy can take more impact, and how to step into the strike and absorb impact so you can control the weapon and stop it. This is covered thoroughly in our intensive weekend trainings. At very advanced levels of training, it is even possible to move with the arc of momentum and almost entirely avoid taking impact while still gaining superior leverage on the weapon. As I mentioned, though, those are advanced skills, and not recommended until you reach that level of expertise. If you are able to, get out of range and run, as you will continue to be out of range, and safe from their attack.

Even with training, when facing a knife, if you do not or cannot get out of range and run, you must understand the reality; you will be cut. When disarming a knife, it is highly unlikely that you will not get cut. There is a lot of fantasy to what you see in the movies and, unfortunately, also in much of the training in many Martial Arts schools when it comes to knives. A person skilled in using them is not to be taken lightly, and if you choose to disarm, you will be cut. The question, then, becomes how are you cut, and where. Even the best techniques and strategies cannot guarantee that you will not get cut, but they can help you to minimize the damage, to successfully disarm, and to make sure you end up in a good position. The best option is to get out of range and run.

Let's talk for a moment about firearms. There are 2 things to consider in firearms the most. If you are going to enter for a disarm, or not. If you are "mobile," meaning you can run, and you are by yourself with no one to protect, that is your best option. Let's discuss why.

Law enforcement has to train regularly with their firearms, and qualify periodically at the range. I consider even the least prepared possible law enforcement officer to be better prepared than the average criminal who may have a gun, because many criminals only have the gun to intimidate, and have not done the training necessary to use a firearm under pressure. If you have ever done any time at a range yourself, you understand the difference between pulling the trigger and squeezing the trigger. There is a correct spot to put your finger so you are able to squeeze the trigger without any effect to the direction and angle of the barrel of the gun. Under pressure, even law enforcement officers, with all their training, often have trouble with this. In fact, I have seen many statistics that say officers only hit the target at "point blank" distance, (10 feet or less), 1 time in 4 in real situations under pressure. How can this be? Firing correctly requires fine motor skill, and we have already covered how this degrades under pressure without lots and lots of experience. So if even law enforcement, with all their training, is only this accurate, how about criminals? I would wager that they are far less accurate. If you can run, I often see people teach to run away in a zig zag pattern to make you difficult to hit, but I would like to say it is better to run in a zig zag that has NO pattern, and look for an opportunity to use cover to change direction if at all possible, like turning a corner around a building. For the sake of definitions, concealment offers no ballistic protection, but doesn't allow you to be seen, while cover offers a physical barrier strong enough to stop ballistics.

If you ARE going to disarm a gun, then you must be much more prepared. The very real possibility exists that you will be shot, so you must be willing to sacrifice your life for theirs if necessary; however, your mentality in the moment must be to survive at all costs, as always in Self Defense. If you do the math and realize you are the one, then you must go for it. At our weekend intensives, we cover the specifics necessary to understand firearms, and what it takes to disarm them. This is not something that I feel I could cover well enough in a book. There are a lot of considerations, and there is a lot of bad information out there from very well-meaning people who are totally wrong. Seek qualified instruction.

Self Defense Mindset: Awareness

Awareness is your number one Self Defense tool. If your awareness is good, you can avoid most potential problems before they become an issue. Another saying we have in Martial Arts "the fastest draw is when the sword never leaves the scabbard, the strongest way to block, is never to provoke a blow, and the cleanest cut is the one withheld." Awareness is what makes all these best outcomes possible.

Awareness of yourself and your surroundings is first. Imagine that you had to defend yourself. Are you sober? Do you have any idea how your skills deteriorate if you are not? You need to be sober to defend yourself well. Are you listening to music? If so, is it quiet and only in one ear so you can maintain good awareness of important sounds around you? What if something happens, and you need to run, are you wearing shoes that have decent tread and support for running? How about your clothes? Are they too restrictive to allow fluid movement? Or are they big and bulky? If someone can easily grasp a handle on you by grasping your clothes, you are not ideally dressed for Self Defense (though at least some of this cannot be avoided). It's more important to understand your possible exposure by the choices you make than anything else.

After you consider your clothing, the next thing to consider is your transportation. Did you plan your route and parking to your destination? Or if you are using public transportation, do you know any transfers you have to take, the route numbers, etc, as they apply to you? If not, you will spend a lot of time being unfocused and distracted, possibly in crowded areas, which exposes you to undue risk. Let's say you have a big event in a couple weeks in an unfamiliar area, but not too far away. You don't want to wait until the day of and then find your way. It's much better to plan it in advance, or even take the route as practice so that when you do it under pressure, you are prepared. Being under pressure, and being in an unfamiliar place, are not an ideal mix.

Next you need to have awareness of the area around you. If you have a family, you may have some of these habits already, such as knowing the location of restrooms in case your family might need one. Do you notice exits? If there is any kind of emergency at all, you might need the exits. If you have medical training, you might notice the signs for AED and first aid stations. If you have ever survived a fire or have fire safety training, you might notice the location of fire extinguishers. If you have military training or have attended an active shooter class, you may notice both cover and concealment, which kinds of doors and windows they are and how they open and close, how they lock, and even the direction they close. I don't advocate being paranoid. Few people need that level of awareness. If you are reading this book, you probably don't. If you need that training, you probably have specific training just for that. But these are some examples. And a little awareness goes a long way. Another chapter has drills that you can use to increase your awareness for Self Defense situations, to make them evaporate almost before they appear.

My last notes on this subject are that if someone is behaving erratically, it would be a good idea to get away from them. Criminals often behave in an irrational manner before they start to commit a crime. If you are in a public place and you get a bad feeling, act on it. Your feelings and instincts are very strong indicators for your survival. Learn how to notice them. If you aren't sure what the signal is, just leave. Change your location. Nearly every time that something major has happened in my life, there was a moment of warning that I ignored.

Many of my Self Defense students have told me that they have felt unsafe and left an area but then nothing happened. They ended up feeling silly that they were "over-reacting." Actually, their taking action, leaving, more than likely prevented the criminal assault from taking place. That, truly, is the best Self Defense, the art of winning without fighting. Better safe than sorry!

Self Defense Mindset: Habits to Cultivate

The most important habit to cultivate if you never want to need to defend yourself is awareness. Simply look up and around you. An enormous number of people do not look around them; they are too absorbed in their phone, their thoughts, etc. Not paying attention like this creates a huge opportunity for a criminal. Your reaction is slowed, so they have much more time to get into position. Look around you. Know who is there. Keep your eyes focused on where you are going, because that creates the ideal leverage to react well.

Prepare before transitions. Let's say you are at the mall and just finished shopping. You take too many shopping bags to your car all at one time, and when you arrive, you look in your purse or pockets for a minute or two for your keys, then you get a text so you check it. Meanwhile, all your stuff is sitting on the ground outside your car while you are distracted. Easy for a criminal to take your stuff, and easy for them to assault you (you are burdened with too much stuff). Instead, if you have 2 people, one could wait inside the store near the doors while the other gets their keys ready in advance, then drives the car up, and picks you and your stuff up curbside. If you are by yourself, when you are buying, you could remember you don't want to carry too much, prepare your keys, and go drop what you've bought so far in your car (cover bags with a blanket so expensive items are not immediately visible), then go back to shopping. If you are heading to a different side of the mall, you could drive your car over to that side so you don't have to walk so far carrying your things, or be sure to walk inside the mall rather than outside. (Thefts still happen inside malls even with cameras. There are blind spots, not all cameras may work, the video may not be sufficient quality, etc.)

Don't linger if you can avoid it. Many people get into their car, and hang out there with their doors unlocked while they do all kinds of things. If you are in darkness or in an area with poor visibility, don't linger. If you have to linger in your car, at least lock the doors. I had heard this but didn't listen. (Tell me and I will forget, show me and I may remember, involve me and I will understand.) I was sitting in my unlocked car once upon a time when an elderly lady with dementia got into my car and started giving me directions like I was a taxi driver. Turned out that she had wandered away from her nursing home, and everyone was looking for her. She had no ID and did not know her name, and the place she wanted me to take her in the cab was in another state. She was only a few blocks from her nursing home, but she didn't know. It took a couple hours to sort out. So glad it all worked out. But what if it had been a criminal instead of a sweet lady who was lost? I was very vulnerable.

Drive with your windows up, and fans on instead of windows down. A few years ago there was a rash of car thefts in my city. Criminals were approaching cars at a stop sign, and poking a gun inside open windows to threaten the driver. All it takes is one person to run across the street, which forces you to stop and visually distracts you leaving you frustrated and off balance, while the other approaches from the side. The criminals never bothered anyone with their windows up, because they weren't good targets.

Do you know the best way to have good visibility around corners? You want to go around them wide, so you have the best visibility possible in advance. If you go tight around the corner, you could unexpectedly find yourself right in the middle of a bad situation.

Plan your route in advance. Because all our smartphones have GPS now, most often when we go somewhere new, we just plug in the address and go. But you may find along the way that you have the street name or number wrong, the city wrong (many identical streets exists in many nearby cities), or the map simply may take you places you would rather not go, or to roads that have changed (the maps are pretty good, but construction happens all the time). If you are in a hurry or are late, you will already be a little on edge, and may not catch every detail right. This can cause you to take the wrong exit, etc, cost you lots of time, or make you lost. If you know you have to go somewhere for something important, consider testing your route in advance so you won't be anxious or late. Preparation is a very smart idea.

Fill your car up with gas. That's right, something so simple is good Self Defense. When you get to halfway, fill up. If an emergency comes up, the last thing you want to deal with is running out of gas. If you do, and you have AAA or some type of emergency roadside assistance, call them if you are in an unknown area rather than leaving on foot. Then while you are alone in an unknown area, call someone and stay on the phone until assistance arrives. Better yet, tell roadside you will be waiting in the restaurant or other public place if it is very close by instead of waiting at your car. If you are going to take care of your car yourself, make sure you keep what you need in your car (flares, reflective signs, wear a reflective vest while you change the tire, flashlight, jack, lug wrench, tire pump, everything you need). Don't drive around on a donut (small emergency tire); carry a full size spare, or put a real tire on ASAP. Ethical tire shops are happy to help you for low cost.

You Cannot Go With Them

You can never go with a criminal for ANY reason. No matter what they may say to you, you cannot go. Don't convince yourself that if you go along now you're just waiting for the right opportunity to go for help later. Don't Go Willingly. Once they have complete control, you may never get control back. To some of you, this may seem like very obvious advice, but I have had this discussion many different times with people who were convinced that the best approach is to "lure them in" to thinking they were in control by just going along, and then make their escape later. I don't know if it's too much TV or what, but somehow this idea persists, and nothing could be more dangerous or wrong.

If a criminal is trying to take you somewhere, it is exactly the place you least want to go in the whole world. THE REST OF THIS SECTION MAY BE SCARY. PARENTS, PLEASE MAKE SURE IT IS APPROPRIATE BEFORE ALLOWING YOUR CHILD TO READ IT. It's much better to fight for your life than to surrender it willingly. It might not only be a matter of life and death, by going along, it might also lead to unspeakable torture. Law Enforcement has a term for the place where a criminal takes you. It's called a 'secondary crime scene,' and it is not a place you ever want to see.

Criminals who plan abductions have scouted out a spot somewhere in advance, and that is where they take you. It's a place they've prepared in advance, and made sure that you will not be easily found, and no one will hear you scream. Very seldom are people found alive at secondary crime scenes in abductions. And there are usually signs that there was extreme physical and sexual abuse while the victim was alive, and sometimes even after they are dead. The people who ARE found alive at these ghastly spots are shadows of their former selves, and desperately need medical attention. When they survive, they are horribly emotionally scarred, and many end up not able to take care of themselves well. Some even take their own lives.

Sorry about that, but you need to know, and if you don't know already, I need to tell you. I don't say all this to scare you, though fear can be a powerful motivator. I say this because I want you to truly understand that YOU CANNOT GO WITH A CRIMINAL FOR ANY REASON. It is better to fight. Even if you are not successful fighting back and you die, that would be preferable than the alternative of a secondary crime scene for many people. At least you died fighting, and not tortured endlessly until you die of dehydration, exposure, or worse.

The problem we get into with this concept is that we all have something larger than ourselves that is more important than our own life. If the criminal convinces us that they will spare a loved one if they can have us, you might consider going along with that. The issue, though, is this: they are a criminal, why would you believe or even listen to anything they say?

I read about a lady who was abducted with her kids. Apparently the criminal told her that if she went willingly, he would leave the kids alone. However, as soon as he got her secured, he went back and got the kids too. When she complained and said that he had promised, he laughed and said, "I'm abducting you! Why would you believe me?" When authorities found her, her children were already dead, and had been tortured terribly. She had been abused in horrific ways and was near death. She rehabilitated enough to get her story out so that we would all know not to listen to a criminal, and about the dire consequences, but she was severely traumatized and scarred. She later took her own life.

I'm so sorry that I have to relay these stories to you. If I knew an effective way to make you understand without having to share them, I would. But I have your best interest in mind. Now that you have read this, you should be prepared and know, if anything ever happens, that you will not go with a criminal, and not listen to what they say.

Weekly mindset training

I have taught a lot of weekly courses where we worked on one particular aspect of our mindset each week, so we would not be a target for criminals. I encourage you to take each of these trainings and practice them for a week. With time, they will become automatic, easy, and will require little effort. I recommend that you do something to prompt you to practice these exercises, such as wear your watch on the opposite wrist, tie a string around your finger, put a rubber band loosely around your wrist, or set an alarm, and whenever you notice the prompt, then you practice the exercise.

The first exercise is to look for exits. If something happens, it is VERY useful to know where the exits are. Running is excellent Self Defense. You might not only save your own life, but if you make a run for it, and others follow you, you might have saved their lives too. When you notice your prompt, look around yourself, and make a quick mental note of all the exits you see. With just a little effort, you will start to do this in everyday situations. Active Shooter classes are popular right now, and this practice should be part of every one of those classes, if they are teaching in the FBI's method of Run, Hide, Fight. If you know where the exits are, you know where to run. I am available to conduct Active Shooter Classes; please ask.

The second exercise is to practice self-awareness. This means that if you understand the things that can make you attractive to a criminal, you turn your attention to yourself and see if you would make a good target. You don't want to go through your day paranoid; remember this is just an exercise, so consider your exposure each time you notice your prompt.

The third exercise is to become aware of criminal opportunities that others present. When you notice your prompt, take a look around you. If you were a criminal, who would you pick out as a target? Look around you and see who is vulnerable and why.

The fourth exercise is to look around and find a person, and practice describing them as if you needed to give the description to the police (instructions on how to do this will be found in chapter 9).

The fifth exercise is to pick out a vehicle and practice giving a vehicle description as if you were doing it for the police (instructions on how to do this will be found in chapter 9).

The sixth and final exercise is to check yourself and others around you whenever you notice your prompt. Are you doing anything that makes you attractive to a criminal? Is someone near you doing something that makes them a good target?

That final exercise is a combination of exercise 2 where you notice yourself, and exercise 3 where you notice others. It is designed to show you how much you have improved since you last did the exercise. Most of my students have found that they have improved dramatically at both minimizing their exposure to casual threats (crimes of opportunity), and identifying risky behaviors that would attract criminals.

It is important to mention again that I do not want you to be paranoid. If you are a civilian, you do not want to go through life on high alert like you would need to if you were in an active war zone. However, developing the skillset for emergency situations is very useful, and highly recommended. Once you have the knowledge, you need only practice very occasionally, and you will be tremendously more protected than before.

Remember that 90% of crimes are crimes of opportunity. If you master these skillsets, the only real concern you have is when you are specifically targeted, the other 10%. For those situations, physical skills are required. Even then, these awareness skills can deflect, defuse, or prevent a good portion of threats by never giving them opportunity to happen.

Chapter 5
College

Statistics

I think statistics are a tricky thing, because I can always find statistics for both sides of any position, so please take these, as any, with a grain of salt; your mileage may vary. These statistics are directly from the website of the college where I have taught so many Kickboxing, Cycling, and Self Defense Classes, Sonoma State University, in Rohnert Park, CA. "Every two minutes, someone in the United States is sexually assaulted...eighty percent of sexual assault victims are under the age of 30...almost two-thirds of victims are assaulted by someone they know...victims are significantly more likely to suffer from depression, post-traumatic stress syndrome, abuse drugs and/or alcohol or to contemplate suicide."

The White House Task Force to Protect Students from Sexual Assault released their first report in April 2014, stating that 1 in 5 college students experiences sexual assault during their college career. Additionally, the ACLU estimates that 95% of U.S. Campus rapes go unreported.

The following statistics come from the National Sexual Violence Resource Center, who provide information and statistics for journalists. 1 in 5 women and 1 in 16 men are sexually assaulted while in college (Krebs, Lindquist, Warner, Fisher, & Martin, 2007). The majority of these crimes (90%) on college campuses are never reported (Fisher, Cullen, & Turner, 2000). Among college women, 9 out of 10 victims of sexual assault knew the person who sexually assaulted them (Fisher, Cullen, & Turner, 2000). In a nationally representative survey of adults,

37.4% of female rape victims were first raped between ages 18-24 (Black et al., 2011). Of the self-reported perpetrators, 75% reported that they had used alcohol prior to their most recent perpetration incident. Incidents involving alcohol were much more likely to include attempted or completed rape than incidents without alcohol (Kingree & Thompson, 2014). Nearly 2/3 of college students experience sexual harassment, and less than 10% of these students tell a college or university employee (Hill & Silva, 2005).

Here are some important things to know about people who commit sexual violence (statistics still from National Sexual Violence Resource Center). About 150,000 adult sexual offenders are currently in state and federal prisons throughout the United States. Between 10,000 and 20,000 are released into the community each year (Center for Sex Offender Management, 2007). More than 700,000 registered sex offenders live in communities throughout the U.S. (National Center for Missing and Exploited Children, 2014). Often, people who sexually abuse are portrayed publicly as "monsters." Because of this, people might be less likely to recognize the warning signs of a sexual behavior problem in loved ones or others with whom they are close, because they do not see them as "monsters." (Tabachnick & Klein, 2011). Once a convicted abuser returns to the community, he/she is subjected to many of the current legislative policies. The resulting housing and job instability, loss of income, and isolation could increase the risk to re-offend. The instability might also reduce the system's ability to monitor the offender and hold him accountable (Tabachnick & Klein, 2011).

From my own experience teaching a few thousand people in the last 20 years, many people are assaulted, and many of them who are, do not want to talk about it, so I believe that all these crimes are very under-reported. Even when victims do report, only about 25% of the time does it lead to any kind of conviction or consequences for the criminal.

The best reason to learn Self Defense is that if you need it, help will not be able to get to you until the situation is all over. No one is going to be able to respond fast enough. You are the first responder. I was attending an active shooter training, and they emphasized how in that situation, you do want to call as soon as you can, but the situations usually resolve before law enforcement has a chance to get there.

Reporting on Campus

One of the main fears that victims face is that the event will become public, and that the person will still get away with it. These fears probably cause the 95% to be unreported (as estimated by the ACLU). Similarly, of what is reported, less than 25% is estimated to result in any legal action against the perpetrator. Actually, given the state of our legal system, perhaps that figure is good. Call me cynical. The important thing to realize is that, if you do NOT report, there is 100% chance that nothing ends up on record, which makes the criminal more likely to both repeat, and escalate. In effect, you doing nothing makes the bad situation worse for the next victim. I know that must be horrible to hear, and I would hate to be in your shoes, but if you are assaulted, I firmly believe it is your responsibility to humanity to report. Everyone is counting on you for their safety. I can totally understand if you cannot, but this decision really hurts everyone, sorry to say.

Now, your college may be different, but here are some ways to report on the campus where I teach: Counseling and Psychological Services, Vice President of Student Affairs, Residential Life Office (for on-campus residents), Student Health Center professional staff (doctor or nurse), any Police and Safety Services Officer. Your campus may have the E-911 technology that places any 911 mobile phone call within the zone to their jurisdiction, though this does not always work perfectly, and you may want to find out the campus number for expediting emergency services at your campus.

The website for my campus is really quite good, nice work SSU, I'm quoting another part:

"Reasons to report a crime include: Reporting within 72 hours... will allow for valuable evidence to be collected. The sooner...the better. Reporting is empowering. It gives survivors... back some of their personal control. Reporting the crime will ensure that medical expenses... may be paid by public compensation funds. Reporting and prosecuting are essential to...protection of other victims by... deterring repeat offenders. Reporting attests... that sexual assault really happens, it is never the survivor's fault, and that the survivor's voice is heard and not silenced. Reporting can help support the case of another survivor... The information you provide might be just enough evidence to...help them get justice."

Consider filing a civil protection order (also called a restraining order). You should not have to be around someone who has assaulted you. (Speak to a lawyer; I cannot give legal advice.)

Confidentiality is a concern for a lot of people, and policies vary greatly by state. Your teachers are likely to be mandated reporters. If confidentiality is a concern, ask their reporting requirements before discussing the situation with anyone. Remember that if someone is sharing your personal and confidential information in this case, they are likely trying to see that you get the help you need. It should be done discreetly and with great care. Medical confidentiality is governed by FERPA and HIPAA. If you have reported at your college and feel that it has not been handled appropriately, contact your title IX coordinator on campus.

There are new online resources:
Itsonus.org – understand sexual assault
Notalone.gov to report sexual assault (includes information for filing with the Office of Civil Rights and U.S. Department of Justice.

Phone numbers:
National Sexual Assault Hotline: 800-656-4673
National Domestic Violence Hotline: 800-799-7233
National Rape hotline: 1-800-656-HOPE

Why college students can be more at risk

College is a big, crazy place. You are busy with 1000 things, trying to find your place in the world, and you don't have enough time to do it all as well as you'd like. In addition to the usual stress of college, more students today than ever before also have to work more hours while they are in school. You are racing around full speed ahead on all cylinders so much of the day, and you will want to blow off steam.

Music can be a powerful way to soothe your emotions, so it is only natural that you would listen to music to control your moods and keep your focus. However, if you are out and about when it is dusk or dark, it is very risky to reduce another of your senses this way. Your vision is already impaired at these times, so it's especially important to have your other senses working for you. At those times, don't have your earbuds in or headphones on. Any time one of your senses is reduced, you will want to be more focused so you can recognize and respond to any changes in your environment. Your hearing can be a great asset for Self Defense.

There's a lot of drama in college life. He said, she said, and all that stuff. It's really not very useful or productive, it robs you of energy, and it can lead you to be very distracted from things that really matter. If you are out in public and are very caught up with and distracted by minor things, you might find yourself in a bad situation before you even realize how you got there. There are a lot of little spots that predators can hide and lie in wait on any campus, and criminals are surprisingly good at finding them.

The statistics are chilling. In nationwide surveys of rape victims, 80% of them were raped before the age of 25, and the majority while they were in college. 50% of rape victims are raped before they are 18. Ladies age 12-17 are 2 to 3 times more likely to be sexually assaulted than adults. Most young people who are sexually assaulted know their assailant. Those who have already been violated before attending college are up to 3 times more likely to be violated again. (I believe this is due to the resulting lowering of self-esteem, depression, and frequent self-medication with alcohol which leaves criminal opportunity. Please do not think that I would ever blame a victim. No one wants to be a victim of a sexual assault.)

The times and locations of sexual assault vary, but the majority occur on late nights and weekends, and off campus at parties where there is alcohol, especially at fraternities. (Ladies who are members of sororities which associate with fraternities at off campus parties are more at risk, as fraternity members perpetrate sexual assault more than non-members.) Ladies in their freshman and sophomore year experience the greatest risk of sexual assault, especially in the first few months of each year.

Set boundaries. Ladies, you have the right to set your boundaries. You have the right to change your boundaries. Don't ever assume that the other person will understand your feelings and thoughts, so be vocal. Never be afraid to say no. Ask for help or make a lot of noise, cause a commotion if you are threatened. It's so much better than the alternative.

If rape happens to you or someone you know, please report it and don't lose any evidence. The majority of rapists are repeat offenders. Gathering evidence should be a huge priority. It can both help catch a criminal, and exclude the innocent, so it is always useful.

Incapacitated rape is a real problem too. If you believe that being drunk enhances your sexual experience, you are more likely to binge drink. And if you binge drink, you are more likely to be incapacitated. Later in this chapter, we'll talk about Self Defense if you are drunk.

Risky Behavior & How to Play It Safe Instead

I quoted statistics earlier that said that 75% of self reported perpetrators were drinking or on drugs during their last sexual assault. It's important to realize how much substances can lower inhibitions for you so you might get yourself into bad situations unknowingly, that you would usually avoid. It's also important to realize how substances can lower the inhibitions of people who might assault others!

I found an article from 2012 about teens on overnight campus visits as part of the selection process for where to go to school. It cites a survey by the Center for Adolescent Research and Education (CARE) and Students Against Destructive Decisions (SADD). Of those who went on an overnight visit, 16% reported drinking during the visit, 17% reported engaging in sex or other intimate behaviors, 5% reported using drugs other than alcohol, and 2% reported driving while impaired. 51% of these teens who reported drinking said they had never done so before. 52% of these teens who reported sexual activity said they engaged in behaviors they previously had not.

Since teens in their first 2 years of college are the most at risk for rape, it makes sense to prepare and protect our youth. Teens, you do not want to be surprised by these situations. Knowing that they may come up allows you to think in advance of what you would like to do, and avoid potentially risky situations. Parents, you cannot completely protect your teen, as much as you would like to do so. If you have open and honest communication, you can ask your teen questions to make sure that they understand the serious consequences that could accompany these poor decisions. If you are reading this book, great! Make sure your teen reads it. Parents, you need your teen to have sources other than you that are authorities that they can listen to and trust. As much as we want to have our children listen and learn, no one likes to be told what to do. Instead, seek to educate them, and encourage them to have mature relationships with other trusted adults (they might ask questions they would never ask of you because you are parents).

A huge percentage of the female college students who drink say that they do it mostly as a means of breaking the ice, having something to do, having a shared experience they can talk about, to allow people to have more fun, creates a connection with their peers, and to facilitate male bonding. Some colleges are getting the message that there needs to be more fun things to do on evenings and weekends right on campus, to provide a safer way to meet all these needs for students without sending them off campus to drink. I know Sonoma State University, where I teach, has added more and more events each year for the past few years for exactly this reason.

There are also frequently intramural sports offered at college, which can provide many of the same benefits of social interaction and friendship building. There are often single gender and mixed gender leagues. I believe these considerations should be part of your selection process of a school. Education is paramount, but you must be happy with your life while you are there in school.

Students, you need to create a peer group that has some classes in common so you have allies who can help you when you run into trouble in a class. Find those people who can help and support you, be respectful, and don't worry as friendships change. As you get along in your major, really get to know the best students.

It comes down to this; you become who you hang around with. If you want to get the most out of your education, you need to spend time with the people who are the most interested in learning.

Self Defense if Drunk or on Drugs

I could spend a lot of time telling you not to drink, and not to do drugs. What I've found, however, is that the more you tell people not to do something, the more they want to do it. So instead, I take a different approach. If you truly understood how amazing you are, and your real potential to have an impact in the world, you would not squander it so easily. You would, instead, go out and live the best life you can for yourself, those around you, and your community. Please realize that I'm not here to tell you how to live your life, and I don't want to even make any kind of value judgments if you are drinking or using drugs. This is not the place for that. My purpose is just to educate you about Self Defense.

Speaking purely from the perspective of Self Defense, then, I can tell you that being impaired in any way is highly risky. If you are going to be doing those things, you need to be in an environment that is totally safe, with people you trust completely. If you are going to be out and about, you must institute a buddy system in advance, with the agreement that you will not leave each other for any reason, and that your buddy has the right to get you home safely, call a cab, not let you leave with someone, etc.

If you are out in public intoxicated, there can be several consequences that can be life altering. If you drink and drive, you could kill yourself or someone else. Even getting a DUI ticket can cause a permanent mar on your record that could prevent you from getting as good a job, etc. It's a really high cost. Don't drink and drive. It's always a better decision to take a cab. Take a cab on the way there to go out instead of driving there so you don't have to leave your car there when you take a cab home.

If you are in public intoxicated, your awareness is almost zero (though it may not feel that way), so you will walk right into situations that you might otherwise easily avoid. If someone overdoes drinking in public and you have to be their caretaker, you are also very distracted, leaving many opportunities for criminal robbery and assault. Keep your drinking light to moderate to avoid this. If you know someone who is participating in these extremely risky behaviors, the likelihood is that they have already been assaulted in some way. People who have suffered assault and suffer from corresponding low self-esteem or risky behavior are often trying to mask the past. When you feel that you are not worth anything, you will make some very bad decisions. No matter what has happened, you are worth it. You are amazing. We need you. Please get help.

Here's the scary part. You need to read this. Criminals are ingenious. In their laziness and selfishness, rather than take time to get to know a woman, honor her, date her, and court her, they have created many different kinds of ways to spike your drink that you would have a hard time detecting. This is such a prevalent problem that there is a company trying to develop a nail polish that can detect the presence of date rape drugs, but they have not had much success, and as of this writing, the company does not have anything available for purchase. This might be because there are so many different compounds that testing is not reasonable. Besides GHB, MDMA, Rohypnol, and Xanax, there are many other compounds that would have the same effect, and many can be bought over the counter (Benadryl, sleep tablets, etc). If a test is ever released, the criminals who make the date rape drugs will just design something enough different to pass the test that still has the same effect. Many of these compounds are clear, so they could even be added to water without visible signs. The only way to be safe with your drink is to make it yourself, and not allow anyone else to come in contact with it.

The biggest consideration for Self Defense is this: If you are impaired in any way, your reactions are incredibly delayed. You may even feel like you are more capable, faster, stronger, etc., but you are not. That perception is just an effect of whatever you are on. In reality, in comparison to a sober person, you are all but helpless. I know that seems really blunt, but it's simple truth. If you are on anything, you may feel sped up, slowed down, mellow, calm, agitated, quick, smart, sexy, all kinds of things. However, to a criminal, you are a perfect target. Unable to notice something is happening until it's too late, unable to offer meaningful resistance, and because you are impaired and will not have clear reliable memory, less credible as a witness (he said she said). We have a new Yes Means Yes consent law in California, but it's not yet clear how much this will really help.

Buddy system

We all know what the buddy system is, right? It's simply when you are not alone, but always with at least one other person. If you are out late at night or going to an unfamiliar area, you're far better off to have someone with you than to be alone. This is not to say that there is no chance of suffering an assault just because you are not alone; it could and does still happen. However, if there are two of you, then you are not as good of a target for many criminals, so you will automatically avoid some. If something happens, since there are two of you, you have a much better chance to fight back well and succeed. With someone else, you have more opportunities to get help. Plus, even if something does happen, a criminal is less likely to spend more time if the odds are not in their favor, so if you fight back effectively, there is an even greater chance of them giving up the attack and leaving. Worst case scenario, you still have two people who might have gotten a good look at a criminal, which might allow for a better description to police.

The buddy system is really genius. It's so simple. Whenever possible if you know you are entering an area that you are not 100% certain about, just have someone with you. Stay together the whole time, and give each other permission to take care of the other should the need arrive (getting them home safely, taking car keys if drunk and taking them home in a cab, etc). This works amazingly well, but only if you apply it. If you start out together and then separate, as so often happens, if you are in a risky situation, you will be alone, without your buddy to help you. Actually, you can prevent many different situations from even developing, simply by having a buddy. Remember that a criminal wants an easy target. So if you and your buddy are both alert and aware, you are not as vulnerable as two people, one of whom is wasted on drink or drugs, for instance. You would struggle to take care of your friend, and a criminal might well take the opportunity. Now, having a buddy is not guaranteed to keep you safe, but two can much more easily defend than just one. Realize that the majority of crimes are not just one person, but 2 or 3, so having a buddy puts you in a significantly better position.

If you should be so unlucky as to suffer a criminal assault, it is very important for your mental health that you avoid being alone for a time. You will likely not feel completely safe when you are alone for a while, and besides this, the sad reality is that criminals very often repeat their crimes against the same victim, usually escalating. This reason alone makes it important for you to follow the buddy system and avoid being alone. If it happened in your home, you may feel much more comfortable staying somewhere else for a while. The simple act of being somewhere else may avoid a repeat attack.

An important part of the buddy system is that you have a specific plan before you go out. You are going to stay together, and be responsible for each other. If you are dedicated to your buddy, and you both view it from the Self Defense point of view, no matter what else may happen, you will understand the value of staying together to help the other get home safe. If you know your buddy well, you might even plan to stay the night together. This way you are more committed, and you know you will plan it to work out that you are together keeping each other safe all night.

Another great idea is to have a third point of contact. Decide in advance a time that another friend will call and check up on you, or a place where you will meet. If you try this method, be reliable about contacting each other and being where you said you will meet. Otherwise your friend may fear the worst when you might just be a little late.

Chapter 6
Parents & Children

Non-Mobile Considerations

We classify you and those you are with as mobile or non-mobile, meaning, you can run away, or that is not a viable option for you. If you have small children, it may not be reasonable for you to just run from danger. They may not run when you tell them, or they may not run fast. In nature, when a predator chases, the slowest animal is dinner. It is no different for us. The criminal wants an easy target, so if everyone but one runs, they will suffer the attack.

If you and your group are mobile (fit, strong adults), then your objective is to break free from any attack and run. As you go, call for help, dial emergency services (9-1-1 in the USA), and make sure that you are safe. Then regroup and make sure everyone is ok, careful to document anything that needs documenting. Consider filing a police report. If this is necessary, everyone should try not to talk about how many people, what they were wearing, etc. Memory is a funny thing, and talking about it together could mess up actual memories with other people's ideas. Witnesses are notoriously unreliable; we all see things differently, and from our own perspectives. But it's better to have your own opinion directly, rather than be confused.

If you are NOT mobile, then you may need to fight. If yelling "Back Off" and other excellent strategies are not working to de-escalate, or you are already under attack, you will have to fight back. One person should call for help and dial emergency services if at all possible. It takes a few minutes at least for help to arrive, almost no matter where you are. By then it will almost certainly be all over, but better to call immediately than not.

If you are already under attack, you must get free immediately, and the person attacking you must realize that you are not one to mess with, so that they will want to disengage, and may even run. We teach a specific strategy to break free from any grip without requiring you to be able to see how or with what hand or at what angle you are gripped. It's difficult to appreciate the value of the technique until you see it in action, in person. I hope I can show you. I could describe it, but it is easy to misinterpret it, and then you might think it will fail. However, it will work 100% of the time against 100% of the people because it is all about using your entire body against a tiny part of the criminal to maximize your own leverage. Children can make it work against adults. Being fit and strong is certainly an advantage always, but we make use of physics to win.

If you are the lone defender (no one else can really help, or everyone else is too young or paralyzed with fear), you must go immediately for the leader. A group of people has a leader, and if the leader is not seen as strong, the group collapses. If you cannot instantly identify the leader, then get the person closest to you. When you take out one, the leader is the one giving the orders and directions to the others.

If you are defending against a group, the worst thing you can do is fall down. One person on the ground against a group standing is no fun. If you are foolish enough to kick, you will likely fall down. When you are on one leg to kick one person, another will need only to lightly touch or bump you, and they can easily knock you to the ground. Kicks are super fun and cool, but highly risky in defending against a group. Kicks sure look good in movies and demonstrations though!

Your response will depend on your training. Without training, the most important thing to keep in mind is that they are fighting for their dinner, and you are fighting for your life, and the lives of your children or group. Be relentless and never give up. Do everything that would be illegal in any kind of sport fight like gouging the eyes. The eyes will not pop out or anything like that (they almost never do except from extreme impact to the side or back of the head with huge blunt force trauma), but the eyes are delicate, and will make a criminal distracted and lower their will to continue. Attacking the head is best because of the effect on the leverage of the attacker. Control the head and you will control the body. If you can't reach the head, get the knees. Knees are incredibly vulnerable. Don't use a fist unless you know how, because it is easy to break your hand. Your palm is actually harder to break. Use that instead.

Avoid wrestling. Remember, this is Self Defense and there are no rules. Wrestling is an awesome sport, but if your body is in a wrestling position, your head and neck are close, allowing access to some of the most powerful targets.

I teach very specific strategies for everything I've just briefly mentioned. Consider learning in person. You'll really get a lot out of it.

Parents, You Cannot Listen & You Cannot Go With Them

I already mentioned a scary story of a woman and her kids. Unfortunately, things like this have happened many times. It happens often enough that you must be certain to learn the lessons so you don't repeat the mistakes. I won't retell the gruesome story from an earlier chapter, but let's examine the problems instead.

There are a lot of lessons to learn here. The first lesson is that you should not even listen to the words a criminal says. Do you understand? They are a criminal. If they say anything, it is designed to fool you, make you hesitate, and serve their agenda only. Once someone starts attacking you or trying to abduct you, you don't stop fighting until you get free and get away. If you have children there with you to protect and running away is not an option, you fight them so hard and so relentlessly that THEY run away. Make lots of noise. It may not make anyone come to your rescue, as many people don't want to get involved, but drawing attention may make the criminal flee.

Remember that a criminal wants an easy target, not an aggressively fighting back target. They are not fighting for their life like you are, they are fighting for their dinner, so to speak. Make sure you follow up with a police report and do your best to provide a description. Criminals often repeat offend, so you might not only save you and yours, but others too. If you are fighting back, you are doing great!

The second lesson is to never give up. NEVER! You might be one moment from driving the criminal away. A motivated parent protecting themselves and their kids is a serious force of nature. If you keep up fighting and making noise, you'll be ok. Actually, the statistics absolutely prove that fighting back is the best strategy. In every case, fighting back helps and doesn't hurt. Fighting back is the only thing that drives a criminal away, never conversation. You cannot talk to and convince a criminal to leave you alone. It simply doesn't work. The psychology of a criminal is that they are trying to put themselves up and put you down. They are trying to dominate and to force you to give in. If you plead with them, "Please leave my family alone," they subconsciously feel powerful and entitled to be doing these bad things. Don't give a criminal that kind of ammunition.

You might actually defuse the situation before it becomes physical if you handle yourself right. If you have your back straight, your head up, and your voice is loud and strong and you say "Back Off!" and "Leave!" you will show a criminal that you are not fooling around. You are NOT the easy target they thought you might be. The right attitude can easily make them find another target instead of you.

The third lesson is that you cannot go with them. If you have thought about this in advance and come to the conclusion, armed with the knowledge of what happens to people who go along with the criminals, that you will not go with them for any reason, then your mind is ready. If your mind will not allow you to go with them, then you will not go. If the worst happens and you die protecting your family, at least you will know that you have done the very best that you could possibly do. However, I really don't think it will work that way. What we find, when we look at all the case studies and the research, is that people who fight back are better off than people who don't, 100% of the time, and that people who fight back often suffer only minor injuries. After all, if you are there with your family, that is quite a bit of work for a criminal. They are counting on you just giving in and giving them whatever they want, and going along quietly. They do not think that you will fight back and be willing to do whatever it takes to survive and protect your family.

What to Teach Your Kids About Strangers

The Polly Klaas Foundation website has an excellent section on strangers. It can currently be found here: http://www.pollyklaas.org /polly-klaas-child-safety/stranger-danger.html. There's also another excellent resource on how to teach kids to be safe without making them scared, https://www.kidpower.org/library/article/safe-without-scared/.

I guess the reason I like these so much is that I teach the same principles. I've never seen these pages before just now, but we're totally on the same page. That's great, because it means that we're all doing what works. Telling your children scary things like how a stranger could take them away and you would never see them again is really not ok. You need a better way to discuss these concepts with your kids, and those links have a lot of great information.

The thing about strangers is that there's a lot of conflicting information for kids. Their parents say not to talk to strangers, but the kids see their parents talking to strangers all day long. Also, children are often victimized not by total strangers, but by people that they know. If you scare kids about strangers, they might think that bad strangers would look scary, but bad people who want to hurt kids go out of their way to look clean and be friendly to lure in children. Instead of thinking so much about strangers, it is far more useful to teach children about behaviors and boundaries. What is OK and what is not. If a boundary is crossed, children need to run away yelling "NO!" as they run, and tell the nearest trusted adult. That adult should contact the parents right away.

Here's a list of behaviors that are absolutely not ok. They require action. Children should be taught to say or yell "NO, LEAVE ME ALONE", and run to tell the closest trusted adult, and this should trigger immediate parent notification. Children should also be taught to trust their feelings. If they start to feel uncomfortable, there is probably a reason.

Here's the NOT OK list
- If someone asks you to keep a secret
- If someone tries to touch part of you that is covered by a bathing suit
- If someone tries to separate you from a group
- If someone you don't know asks for your help (you are a kid, you can help only with your parents nearby and with their instruction. Lots of predators use the "help me find my lost dog" to start conversations with children and lure them away
- If someone you don't know tries to get you to come to their vehicle (needing directions, cool car so take a ride)
- If someone tries to give you food, snacks, or drinks without your parent's permission

Things to teach your kids
- Their first and last name
- Parents' first and last names (you would be surprised how many children do not know their parents' names, only mom and dad)
- Parents' phone numbers

Parents, make sure your emergency contact numbers are kept up to date with school, sports, etc. At school, if they are having trouble, they need help from their teacher, playground supervisor, crossing guard, office staff, principal, nurse, whoever is closest. It's important that your child know that if they don't feel safe, they always have permission to call or reach you and that you will come help them. If they tell one adult and it is not resolved, they need to tell another one or you right away. Follow through and make sure it is resolved for your child's safety.

It's also important to teach children how to identify strangers who can help them. Policemen and firemen in uniform are a good example of good, trusted strangers. If your child gets separated from you and lost, everyone they see will be a stranger. Who will help them? They need to know who to go to. If they are lost in a department store, they can go to any counter that has a cash register, walk right behind the counter to the cashier, and say that they are lost and need help. I'm confident that the cashier will be able to page security and get them help. If a child is lost on the street and there is a shop nearby (coffee shop, restaurant, or someplace with lots of people), they should do the same thing; go inside, go right behind the counter or at least directly to the front of the line and say they need help because they are lost. Your children need to have some form of identification bracelet with important medical information, especially when they are young, and this can easily be made to include ways to contact parents.

Children need to know that you love them unconditionally, no matter what. They need to feel safe to tell you things, and that you will make everything OK and always love them. Sometimes a predator can convince a child that it is the child's fault, and their parents would be mad at them. Make sure your kids know they can tell you anything and you will always love them. It is useful to have your children rehearse the NO and LEAVE ME ALONE response. Without practice, they might freeze, or might not remember what to do.

When you are out and about with your kids, you could periodically ask them if there was an emergency, who would be good to ask for help? Is there a friend nearby? Who nearby could be a safe stranger? Don't overdo it; a little goes a long way.

Self Defense For Children

There's almost no difference between what I teach children physically and what I teach adults when it comes to Self Defense. Our concepts are designed to be used by someone smaller and weaker against someone bigger and stronger, so they work well for kids and adults alike.

The part that IS different is that I emphasize more what children need to say. If someone is trying to abduct a child, I teach them to yell NO and HELP, I DON'T KNOW THEM! I can't just teach kids to yell "You're not my mom/dad" because there are so many families with step-kids (I am a step-dad), and some kids will say that exact phrase. I got in the middle of a mom and daughter once because the daughter was screaming bloody murder that "You're not my mom!" in a mall. Turned out that the mother was a step-mom, and the child was young and having a really bad day. It was awkward for everyone that I got involved, and maybe I shouldn't have, but I just had to be sure the child was ok. I ended up asking the young child to please say things like "I don't want to go" and find better words, explaining that "You're not my mom" made me think she was being stolen by a bad person. If that mother ever reads this, I hope she will forgive me; I really did mean well. I'm very sorry. When it comes down to it, I'd rather make sure a child is safe, no matter the awkwardness.

The problem that kids could easily run into is that passive onlookers, everyday busy people, could just think that they are a misbehaving child and the parent is struggling to find the right way to deal with them. We all instinctively pay less attention in that type of situation because it is not our place to get involved, and we want to give the parent the privacy necessary to get their child to be calm and well-behaved. I actually think there's a big problem with parents allowing spoiled behavior in their children, because if children learn that it is OK to act up like that without consequences, it makes it hard for other adults to distinguish between a situation where they need to intervene (abduction), and just bad behavior. Speaking of bad behavior, I was a very unruly and badly behaved child. Possibly because I was overly curious, didn't listen and obey well, and incredibly loud. I don't know how my parents dealt with me; I was a real pain. Thanks for raising me Mom and Dad!

I think the very best thing for children is to learn Martial Arts. I teach Karate to kids, and I think that's the best thing for them, but you have to find the right teacher in your area. Kids benefit from structure, so they need to study an art that has a belt system with increasing challenges as you work your way along. Whether Karate, Taekwondo, Judo, Kung Fu, or some other art, they will benefit immensely if you find the right teacher. The teacher should have a lot of experience with kids, and their philosophy should be similar and complementary to your own. I use positive praise and point out positive examples whenever possible rather than NO and DON'T and BAD or WRONG. I like to catch someone doing something good and praise it. Everybody likes praise. Nobody likes to feel bad. Kids need lots of positive role models of other kids their own age, older kids, and adults. Parents, as much as you want to, you can't teach your own kids everything yourself. You're going to have to find other people that you like and respect, and allow them to mentor your kids. Otherwise, your kids will find other people that you might NOT like, and emulate them instead.

But the great thing is that there are all different kinds of people. My approach may not be compatible with yours. Find a teacher whose philosophy on correcting children is similar to your own, or one that you would like to use. Parents in my school often use tips they learn from me. I have picked up MANY tips from parents and everyone else who I saw doing anything that worked. That's my secret to excellence. Always be learning, and everyone can be your teacher.

Strategies Criminals Use to Abduct/Victimize Children

Child abduction is not the huge and common crime you might imagine it to be in the USA. It accounts for only about 2% of crimes against children. The majority of those cases are Parental Child Abduction (discussed below). Some cases are acquaintance abduction, where the child knows the person somehow. Least common are stranger abduction. However, it does happen, however uncommon, and human trafficking and child sexual abuse also happen (discussed below).

Even though child abduction is not common, criminals do use strategies to lure and victimize children. This is frightening stuff, but important to learn. Here are some strategies criminals commonly use:
- Asking a child to help them find their lost dog/cat (they may even have a printed flyer of the animal for 'proof')
- Driving slow around a neighborhood in a fancy/cool car, and if a child sees it and approaches, asking the child if they want to take a ride
- They will start with offering some small gift, and if the child and parent accept it, they will slowly do more and more for the child. This will seem that they are building goodwill, but why? Be careful with people who are too eager to help.

At a Martial Arts tournament I was attending as a judge, I once got a really creepy feeling from someone. He was helping as a volunteer. A very large and obese man, he was out of place at a Martial Arts tournament. I told my students to stay away from him at all costs because I trust my instinct. My good friend, another instructor, also got a creepy feeling. We decided to complain to the tournament promoter, saying that we got the feeling he should not be allowed around children, and had he been background checked, etc? (I am now part of USA Karate, which requires all coaches and referees to be Background Checked, CPR certified, and Safesport Certified by the United States Olympic Committee, but this group had no such protections.) The tournament promoter told me that this guy was an old student of his who liked to help out around the school and events, and was always helping families, picking up kids from school, taking them to appointments, etc. I asked "Why does he do this?" The promoter did not know, but said that the guy was not married and he assumed he always wanted kids. A couple years later I heard from the promoter and he explained that it was discovered the creepy guy was molesting children. The promoter was helping to prosecute him to the fullest extent of the law. If you are a Martial Arts instructor, coach, or work in a school, make sure to do fingerprinting and background checks for all your staff, for anyone that works with kids. It's only good sense, and in many places, it's the law.

Please don't teach your children that strangers look and act scary. This could be true, but quite often, people who actually hurt children go out of their way to look clean and act appealing to children. If you teach them that strangers look and act scary, they won't recognize a true bad person. Teach them instead about unacceptable behaviors, as previously discussed.

Missing & Exploited Children

Unfortunately, human trafficking and child sexual abuse are a real problem.

Website for the National Center for Missing & Exploited Children, www.missingkids.com

24 Hour Hotline if you think you have seen a missing kid 1-800-THE-LOST

Parental Child Abduction

I would be remiss if I didn't include small mention of this, though this area is outside my expertise. However, parental child abductions are far more common than stranger abductions. It happens when one parent wants to circumvent the decision of a court regarding custody. Congress has enacted many civil and criminal laws to address abductions, kidnapping, interstate and international child custody and visitation disputes. If a child is missing and there is a non-custodial parent, the authorities will probably consider them as a suspect first. This does not imply guilt, but it happens so often that they have to be sure.

How to Handle Bullies (another upcoming book)

This is actually a very big subject. I have done a lot of work here, and I have a lot of thoughts on the subject. I am available to visit your group or school to lecture on bullying. Everyone who has attended my bullying events has gotten a lot out of them. I will probably write a book on bullying down the road, but here are some notes for you for now.

Bullying has gained a lot of attention in the last few years, and there are now more resources than ever to combat and learn about bullying. The best website, I feel, is this one: http://www.stopbullying.gov/

If your child suddenly has behavior issues or no longer wants to do a favorite activity, your first thought should be bullying. Bullying takes many forms, and can be very subtle, but it is all hurtful. Bullies have frequently been bullied themselves at home, or have seen bullying behavior modeled, and seen the bully get what they want. Feeling powerless, they often bully others smaller or weaker so that they can regain some feeling of control and power. It's a horrible vicious cycle. Bullying is usually not about the victim. It is about the bully, and their bad feelings about themselves. They feel inadequate (they may be told they are inadequate), or they have a feeling of powerlessness and they are trying to feel strong. The only way they know how is to do the same to others that has been done to them. In a Self Defense book, however, we cannot think too much about the bully. Let's leave that for the professionals who work with child psychology. If this is your profession, you need to know the signs and what to do to help those kids.

The best way to avoid being a victim is to have good self-confidence. If you have a strong sense of self-worth, you will know that you deserve to be treated well. If a bully treats you poorly, you will set a boundary. If the bully crosses the boundary, you will leave the area and report it rather than have a physical confrontation (in school these days, both people are usually punished whenever things get physical. School administration expects you to just leave if you are really being bullied).

Bullies always pick on weaker targets. Someone who they think will not resist, complain, report, or even react except by shutting down or allowing the behavior. If you see bullying behavior, you need to stand up to it, and say "Leave them alone!" Standing up to bullies doesn't stop with just saying No to the bully. You also need to report bullying that you witness. Witnesses are very powerful, and this is a very important responsibility. Not saying anything sends the message that the bullying is ok, to the bully, the victim, the other students, and the school. Be strong. Stand up for others, and stand up for yourself.

If a Bully Gets Physical

If a bully puts their hands on you, you have the right to defend yourself. Fight back, never give up, and look for the opportunity to run. Go directly to the yard duty, teacher, school administration, coach, or principal, whoever is the closest and most appropriate. Get your parents involved. You will need to document what happened in case it happens again. A paper trail is extremely important to protect you and your child. It is possible that your child will still get suspended if they fight back. It depends on the school policy. Make sure that you document whatever happens, as you may need it later. Keep good records.

If consequences are not severe enough for the bully, they tend to go bigger and bigger. Stop them in their tracks by making consequences strong. Personally, I would go all the way to a police report if someone got physical with my child. This way, there is a paper trail, and it puts the bully and their parents on notice that there are consequences. This is not only for your child, but for the bully too. If they learn that actions have consequences early enough, they may change before the bullying habits become so ingrained.

Someone I know well was being bullied, and they reported to their school many times, even to the on-campus police. The police talked to all witnesses, but the witnesses were either friends of the bully or afraid of the bully, so the police did not find out what really happened, and he did not file a report. Because there were not consequences, the bully escalated and got more physical with the same lack of consequences. Finally after several times of escalation, it became both a physical and sexual assault because it happened in the locker room amongst children who were not fully dressed. Still there were no consequences, so the parent realized they would not get the help they needed from the school, because somehow, things were being confused there. They brought the complaint to their local police department, filed a police report and a complaint, and things seem to have improved. The next step would have been to hire a lawyer. If you are not powerful enough to make a bully stop, go one step up the chain until you find a consequence that will stick. (I am not advocating violence.) Even a counselor was involved, but did not help the situation. I personally feel that the bully needs to face sexual assault charges, have time in juvenile hall, that the school needs to be fined, and the parents of the bully need to face fines and jail time. I am probably way too close to the situation to be objective. The victim was not upfront with their parent about what happened and how severe it was the first time, because of embarrassment. This victim mentality enabled the situation to go from bad to worse. By the time the parent realized what was really happening, it was quite severe. You are your own best advocate. Stand up for yourself the first time. Do not allow escalation. Be sure it is handled all the way through until there are consequences, and it does not need to escalate. I was bullied as a child, and the same thing happened to me. This is certainly why I react so strongly to the whole situation. I did not have the skills then to deal with it, but now I do, so I hope you will learn the easy way rather than the hard way. Teach your children to be strong and stand up for themselves, and make sure they get the help they need, and keep asking until it is taken care of!

Chapter 7
Physical Techniques

Limitations of a book

The truth is, a book is very limiting on what it can teach you about physical techniques. A picture, even a series of pictures, is not enough to do much for you. Hearing about a concept is fine in general, but not for a physical technique. Seeing a physical technique can make you think you understand it, but there might be a lot more going on that is not easily visible unless you have spent a long time studying Martial Arts and already have a high level of skill. What I am saying is this: You truly need hands on experience with someone qualified to teach you. I offer introductory and intensive training workshops, so if you are interested in learning directly from me, you certainly can. If you want to find someone close to you for ongoing learning, I will help you with that too. Another later section of the book is all about how to continue to learn based on your goals, needs, and desires.

I have a website, www.immediateselfdefense.com. It is far better than nothing, but all I can do with it is SHOW you some limited concepts, you cannot FEEL them applied to you and know that you are applying them correctly. It's completely different to talk about something than to try it in real life, as I'm sure you know. However, if you were to pay careful attention and practice with a partner following my instructions on the website, I'm sure you could get something out of it, or I would not have taken the time, energy, and gone to the expense to have made training videos available.

As far as in a book, there are a few things that we can talk about and describe as far as physical techniques. We will do that in the next few pages. They include:

- Targets – where should you focus your attention and why
- Drills vs. Static Training – why do both exist? What are their purposes? What should you do?
- Working With Instincts – what is natural to your body? How do you use that?
- Ideal Leverages – what is mechanical advantage as it relates to using your body?
- Adrenaline & Pressure – what changes under pressure? What does that mean for Self Defense?

Advantages of a Book

Actually, a huge percentage of people reading this book will never set foot in a class or try anything hands on in any way. For many different reasons, some people will not pursue physical training. The advantage of a book, then, is to reach that audience, and try to give them the most important skills that I can through a book, training their mindset. If they understand that they are important, that they deserve to live in peace without fear, how to avoid a criminal, and so on, they are a huge step ahead.

An Uncomfortable Truth

I have met people who have attended my lectures (I frequently lecture to introduce a series of physical courses), who are very likely to need to defend themselves at some point because of a visible physical limitation (such as walking with a cane, having a deformed spine, being in a wheelchair, etc). Sometimes, when I encourage them to attend the hands-on class, they feel that there is nothing they could do, so why bother. It's not true. You can become a harder target. If you have a limitation like these, you really should learn how to adapt your body to Self Defense (what works for you). If you don't, and something does happen, you might be helpless to prevent it. Criminals look for easy targets. If you look like an easy target, the chances they will target you are that much higher. If you prove that you are a hard target, no matter what you may look like, they are that much more likely to leave you alone.

My Friend Steve

My friend, Artist and Renaissance Man, Steve Brummé, had polio as a child, (not so common anymore, thank you Rotary!), and gets around on crutches (and a hand-pedaled bike, but that's a story for another time). He loves Martial Arts and has studied for probably 20 years now. He might appear to be an easy target, because he is usually on crutches, but he is absolutely not. Nobody messes with Steve, and if they do, they learn real quickly not to. You don't have to spend so long just to learn basic Self Defense; Steve just does it because he loves it so much. Everyone should learn some Self Defense, especially if there is something that would attract a criminal to choose you as a target.

Targets

Where you choose to target your efforts is incredibly important. Targeting the wrong places will not allow you to be effective. The single biggest mistake that people make in targeting is not realizing how much people move. If you want to train accuracy on a small moving target, it is quite a process. You have to consider your own body mechanics, the angular momentum of your movement (straight line or curve), and how is it possible for the target to move so you can practice for different contingencies. I hope I have illustrated how difficult this can be. Add to this that you should also be in motion so you keep your balance.

Before we discuss targeting, we need to discuss what we call body weapons. These are parts of your body that can be used as weapons for Self Defense. Although the fist can be incredibly strong when it is trained, there is no injury more common than a broken hand in Self Defense when untrained people try to punch. My advice is NOT to use the fist if you haven't been trained how. The palm is a much better tool for most people. The forearm just in front of the elbow, and the back of the arm just past the elbow are great tools. Using the tip of your elbow is to be avoided because if you break that part, you will have a hard time using your arm. The correct spot just above your knee is also a very strong weapon, but it should only be used for certain targets. Don't raise your leg too high, or you risk falling down, something we do everything we can to avoid.

Our primary targets are the eyeband (everywhere glasses would cover including the nose, and all around the head at that height, including the sides and back of the head), the groin, and the knees. That's it! There are certainly lots of other great targets, but they move a lot, and take more training to use. The majority of the trunk (chest, sides, and back), are really not effective to try to target for untrained people (trained people can make use of extremely powerful points like the solar plexus, liver, and kidneys). Under the stress of a real situation, fueled by adrenaline, most of these attacks by untrained people are not effective, land off target, and slide off without being effective. Instead, we are targeting the criminal's posture so he's less effective, and his most vulnerable targets so we can stop him and get away. Many people teach you to attack the throat, and that can work well, but I've found untrained people get better results targeting the eyeband because of the resulting effect on the criminal's balance and ability to continue to attack.

Here are our essential rules. Palms are to be used when you are at greater range, to the head and face, especially around the eyeband (everywhere that glasses would cover). Palms are to be used to the groin in a whiplike motion or a grab (a strong strike doesn't overstimulate the nerves the same way a whip or grab does) when you are closer. The top of your knee (right above the kneecap) is to be used on the outside of their legs (there is a branch of the sciatic nerve in the middle of the leg which is close to the surface and very accessible). It will make a tall person buckle over and come down to a manageable height. It can also be used on the inside of the knee, which almost certainly results in an injury, and will likely prevent them from being able to chase you well as you run away. Forearms and elbows are to be used at close range. If the person is tall you strike the groin or use your knees as described, then they are down to your height and you can use forearms and elbows to strike the head. The head is best struck by the forearm while supported on the opposite side by the palm. Surround the head and strike it so force transfers correctly. All traditional styles of Martial Arts include this technique as a mainstay of Self Defense.

All of this is easier to understand in person, of course. I offer lots of opportunities to learn with me in person if you are interested. Also, if you got this book at the recommendation of another Martial Arts or Self Defense teacher, they can probably show you what we are talking about here. Kudos to them for promoting something they didn't write themselves – we probably think along very similar lines, and I hope this book is useful for them and their students. Actually, I looked for a long time for a book that I could use to supplement my own teaching instead of writing one, and I just didn't find one that I liked. They were either too long, too complicated, or went off in weird directions that weren't useful for the kind of average people that I mostly teach Self Defense classes for.

Static Training, Drills, Dynamic Training

I am defining static training as anything where there is not dynamic whole body movement all the time. Static training with partners with pre-defined limited responses is a very useful way to introduce new concepts. This way you can understand the concept in its pure form, uncluttered by extraneous details. You can work with small or large amounts of resistance, as static training is tightly controlled, and lends itself easily to these adjustments. In static training it is safe to learn to work with the actual targets you would use in Self Defense, and to see how the body would react in an abstract way. Working with them at speed would almost certainly result in injury. In fact, the way our techniques work, wearing armored suits only provides limited protection.

However, in real life, things happen incredibly quickly, and it would be foolish to only do static training. You must apply more and more speed and variation with time. It is when you apply more speed and more variation that you will find your training breaks down if it is insufficiently developed or too complicated for you to presently use. And this is without even considering adrenaline and the pressure of real life circumstances, which degrade your skills an unimaginable amount.

To bridge the gap between static and dynamic training (discussed later), we have drills. Drills are when you take the concept in the abstract (static), and apply it to multiple different directions, adding an additional common variation at the beginning or the end of the concept. You might also drill with more than one person, but at a slower than normal pace while you are learning. Drills are not as clean and perfect as static training, but they allow you to deal with a concept in a much more realistic way, while you are still developing your skill. It is important to realize that all forms of practice, static, drills, and dynamics are important to review, and should always be part of your arsenal of skills.

Dynamic training takes a couple different forms. You can have a cluster of related prescribed attacks from your attacker and practice dealing with them. You can have more than one attacker doing prescribed attacks in sequence so you train your brain to jump quickly from one engagement to the next. You can have one attacker with a set attack with an additional attacker or two without their attack set.

This is an amazing form of training, and you are never too good to practice this way.

The thing that all good training requires is trust and control. Because we are not studying sport fighting, but real life Self Defense, the targets we use and the way we use leverages are highly dangerous at speed and with power. We must moderate ourselves carefully to avoid injury, while still allowing a high level of realistic training. This is a fine balancing act. The best way I've found to work like this is with a small group of people in intensive training over several days. This way we can all learn to trust each other, and how to control our techniques. Injuries should be avoided at all costs.

A book is really very limiting in an ability to get these concepts across. You are invited to visit our website, www.immediate selfdefense.com, to engage in live training events, and encouraged to find a teacher near you who trains in this way. My best advice in however you choose to practice is to get competent instruction, and always pay attention to your posture. You want your back straight, and your head back so it is not a good target. Using a wrestler's shooting posture is a terrible idea in real Self Defense, because in real life the eyes and eyeband are powerful available targets. Strikes to these areas are forbidden in sports, and for good reason. Likewise strikes to the groin and knees can cause tremendous amount of pain and even permanent injury, so training must be controlled.

Working with Instincts

Every living thing has instincts. Instincts are powerful, and they serve important functions. It is instincts that make us pull our hand away if we touch a hot burner on the stove. Instincts are useful, and no matter how far we go, we do not want to totally abandon our instincts, they are too deeply embedded.

Instead, in Immediate Self Defense, we work with understanding what our instincts are, and why. Everyone has certain things that our nervous systems are designed to do. We are truly not that different from one another. We will react in certain predictable ways because we are designed to. As we understand HOW we actually react, we can then understand that since we know we will react that way, what are the techniques and strategies that lend themselves naturally to those reactions?

By working with the body's natural instincts, we are instantly effective. We don't have to take a long time learning how to do something and thinking of what to do in different situations. Instead, we obey certain basic principles of body mechanics, and do what comes naturally. Rather than ever trying to fight the flow of adrenaline, we embrace it and use it to our advantage, being mindful of how it affects us, and learning to recognize the feeling and effects it produces for us.

By contrast, often in Martial Arts, we make use of total body reprogramming to give you ideal responses to every possible scenario. This total rewiring changes many of your fighting instincts. However, with insufficient training, you are left without access to your natural instincts, and with insufficiently developed new instincts. This is part of what creates confusion and a freeze response for some "experienced" people. If they had sufficient experience, they would have trained past this, but without enough training, they may get stuck in a dangerous repetitive loop.

Adrenaline and its effects is not usually accounted for in Martial Arts until you are more advanced, because frankly, it is difficult to do, and requires small groups and lots of trust. It is awkward and counterproductive to try to teach this to a large group of people, or ones who you don't have a good trusting relationship with. In advanced Martial Arts, you can do more of this training more safely, because you will have built the necessary foundation to do it the best way possible.

Self Defense training makes a good foundation for Martial Arts training. You would then already have good responses for effective defense, and can work on improving your reactions. This is also why I say that you should not study Martial Arts if you will not devote at least 2 or 3 hours a week for at least 5 years. It is unlikely that without this basic level of competence, you will have changed your nervous system to a better way, and instead, may be a bit of a mess when it comes to function.

However, taking the long view, a fully trained martial artist can deal nearly without effort with almost any number of people hand to hand. Seems crazy, right? But I frequently demonstrate this to groups. You simply cannot get enough people close enough to stop a trained person. You all get in each other's way. Frankly, once you get beyond about 3 people, you are less effective in a group.

Ideal Leverages

There is an ideal way to use your body to do anything. Most people do not use their body in the ideal way, and this is why both acute injuries and chronic injuries are so common. If you use ideal posture the majority of the time, injuries can be greatly reduced. You want the body to be able to work as the body is designed to work. You need proper posture so that the bones can do the job of holding your body in position. If you are holding a bad posture, your body will do it, but it will do it by making the muscles work hard to hold the posture. That is not the job of the muscles. The skeleton supports your weight and basic position, while the muscles expand and contract to make you move and transfer power. If your muscles are being used just to hold yourself in position, that means they have less expansion and contraction available to make any movement. This, of course, means the movement will have less than ideal strength and power. I know this is a very simple concept and it seems completely self-explanatory, but I cannot tell you how often I see people using unusual postures, saying they are useful for Self Defense. If you give up full functioning of your body, and lose potential power, that is not useful. When you use a strange position, you also slow down your reaction speed and ability to move out of the way and adapt to changing conditions. This is a huge problem. If you have improper posture, your breathing can be greatly affected too. Without good breathing, you will soon find yourself totally out of breath, which is highly dangerous in a Self Defense situation.

For some reason, many people who think they know how to defend themselves will adopt a posture where they hunch over low with their head up and their hands up. Perhaps they've watched a lot of fighting sports on TV or even participated with fighting sports such as wrestling. They might say they are about to "ground and pound." If you are defending yourself and you ground and pound, what if there is a second attacker? You are still sitting down (even though you are on top of someone punching them); can you defend yourself well against an additional standing person or two? Fighting sports are not Self Defense. This is not to say that there are not great skills to be learned, but they must be a little different to apply to a Self Defense situation. When teaching hands-on classes, I always have a couple people who do this. Usually they have some kind of a fighting sport background, and often, they think of this posture as ideal Self Defense. This is a terrific posture for sports, depending on the rules, and terrible for Self Defense. Often the people who show me these postures have less than 5 or 10 years training. It's not that their arts are at fault and don't contain the real solutions to Self Defense problems. As I've mentioned earlier, I like ALL the Martial Arts. I've tried as many as I can, and found them all excellent. Instead, the problem is that the students didn't study enough, and didn't learn the difference between sport with rules that limit targets, and life or death Self Defense. Sometimes, perhaps the people who taught them were not really qualified teachers, unfortunately. There are a lot of people teaching now who were not students long enough and did not get enough depth of experience.

If you are doing a fighting sport that does not allow strikes to the temple, medulla (back of the head), and eyes, then it is nothing like real life or death Self Defense. They must not allow those targets for sport fighting, or there would be too many deaths. You can do great drills by limiting targets and controlling the action, but realize that they are just drills, ways to train to work on specific skillsets, not realistic Self Defense. In Self Defense we use ONLY the targets that are not allowed for sport fighting. They are the most effective. Why waste time with anything except what is so dangerous that you can't allow it in sports? You want your Self Defense training to be effective IMMEDIATELY.

This next paragraph is for Martial Arts teachers who are teaching Self Defense. I hope you will take my advice and benefit from my experience. It has been hard-won. Whenever I teach Self Defense and someone uses postures like this or tries to use them with me, I praise them for their experience and show them how to apply what they know to real life. I show them how their posture is perfect for the rules of their sport, and how dangerous it is when there are no targets prohibited. I explain how and why strikes to their exposed areas work and how leverages work on their head and neck, and then let them experience the difference of superior posture and footwork to their sport posture. I do it in a very friendly, non-confrontational way, and I try to pull them off to the side and do it in private rather than in front of the group. If you have been teaching for a while, you will recognize that someone has this kind of background, and rather than embarrassing them or creating a confrontation where you will have to hurt them to help them understand (I've made both of these mistakes and have finally learned a better way), follow my advice. Praise them. Honor them for their training. If you've done their arts, even better; you can mentor them as a senior with more experience.

If not, don't worry; you can still help them to see things clearly as they are instead of through the lens of sport. Just handle the situation carefully. You don't want the big problems that can come from just beating them up. If you are teaching, you should not need any ego gratification. You should be past that. It's quite easy to hurt people; it's quite another to educate them, and mentor them instead. Some people just need to feel and see the difference, and they will understand. Just let them know that what they do is perfect for certain situations, but then put them in another situation and open their eyes. They ground and pound one. Two others are standing and striking them or manipulating them. Don't they wish they were standing and could move? They have more options if they are standing.

You will occasionally find someone who will not be convinced that their way is not the best. It's hard for them because what they do has worked for them or they believe that it would. Best to just put them with a partner who will enjoy working that way, and keep the two of them light and friendly. Don't allow them to hurt someone. People with something to prove are often the most aggressive. If nothing else works, ask them to leave. I have not been in this position, but I would refund any unused portion of their tuition, or perhaps the whole thing. I have had people consider studying with me that I didn't think would mesh with my student body. They are welcome to private lessons as I am quite adaptable and don't have a problem with anything, even "tough" or "challenging" questions and behavior, as long as it is done respectfully and privately. Not every teacher can teach every person, especially in a group environment. It's ok! That's why there are so many different arts, styles, and teachers. Let them find the right place for them.

Adrenaline & Pressure

If your Self Defense plan does not consider adrenaline, or gives it inadequate attention, it really will not serve you well. Far too many people teach and try to follow very complicated strategies that require precision work and fine motor skills. These skills are almost completely lost under the effects of adrenaline. When your blood pressure spikes so dramatically and your breath begins to change, you lose any real possibility of having accuracy on fine detail work with your hands.

Actually, I think we are all familiar with adrenaline. If you have ever had to speak publicly, you may have felt the rush and nerves, sometimes shaking that can come upon you. This is a result of adrenaline and its effects on the body. If you've ever had someone shout in your face and your blood began to boil, you have felt adrenaline then too. If you've been in an accident you may have experienced the effects of adrenaline.

When we work with adrenaline and pressure, we work with pressure first. Adrenaline work is more advanced, and requires a lot of trust. Just working with pressure will trigger a bit of adrenaline, so it is the perfect warmup to advanced training.

There are two ways to work on pressure and adrenaline – the long road and the short road. The long road is ideal, but it takes several years minimum, or focused training. Using the long road, you work on lots of safe, fun ways to work with pressure and adrenaline. You do sparring and drills in various ways with various methods to expose you to the concepts, and you periodically speed them up and put them under pressure to test how much your training has penetrated your nervous system. You gradually combine all the different methods of training and work in a more and more realistic way. This is the Martial Arts way to train. Slow and steady wins the race, and leads to the very best results.

The short road is for people who have less time to devote to training. It is the Self Defense course method. This is for people who want to feel and be safe, and don't have years to devote to training.

Instead, we teach you just one or two concepts that are natural to your body, and put you under pressure repeatedly. This way you will train past the freeze response. Most people will want to stop if they do the wrong thing. Understand this well. There is NO wrong thing to do, as long as you start moving and keep fighting. You will discover how easy it is to do SOMETHING, and all you need to truly defend yourself is to have ANY response, and just keep on fighting. Fight and fight and never give up. Remember, a criminal wants an easy target, not one that fights back and never gives up.

Actually, I would prefer that all my Martial Arts students go through the Self Defense course method too, then they will get more out of their Martial Arts training, and they will appreciate it more. Martial Arts offers lots of benefits beyond those from Self Defense.

We have to be compassionate when we work with adrenaline. More people than you realize have had different forms of trauma in their life. Often, the trauma will come bubbling to the surface. In the moment of Self Defense, they must train right through it, but when it is over, they may need compassion. They may want to talk, they may not. They may want to be alone (but someone should be nearby in case they need anything). They may want to run away (though you should not let them if they are not safe to do so. Instead, find them a quiet place to gather themselves). Have tissues and water and crackers on hand. Seriously. You need compassion if you do this work. People who have faced trauma may have to experience those feelings many times to feel safe.

Even if a person has NO trauma, working with adrenaline is a bit traumatic itself (that's why it triggers thoughts from traumatic life events). That doesn't mean it is bad or should be avoided. It means that you need special skills to work safely in this way. When adrenaline runs out, you will experience a crash. You will need to rest and recover a bit. Most people feel amazing after they have worked with adrenaline, and find it a life-changing experience.

Chapter 8
Self Defense Tools

False Sense of Security

I see a lot of people who teach Self Defense, and an even greater number of people who do not teach Self Defense but advocate for personal safety in different situations, stressing the importance of Self Defense tools. This is really important, and I need to address it.

Self Defense tools have the potential to be very helpful, if you feel like you might need it so you get it ready and carry it at the ready. Actually, this is what I teach with a tactical flashlight if it is dark outside. Before you transition into an area with poor visibility, you get your tactical flashlight (extremely bright flashlight that will blind someone) ready, and carry it high in your non-dominant hand. This is the equivalent of a police officer's low ready position with their gun. The time-consuming part of gripping and unholstering is avoided in a confrontation.

If you have a Self Defense tool with you, but it is not available immediately, you might have felt safe because you bought it, but if you did not bring it and do not have it at the ready, you have a false sense of security. My biggest issue with Self Defense tools and the way they are marketed is that people can come to rely on the tool instead of learning real Self Defense.

If you don't have the tool with you when the situation comes up, it is useless. If you do not have it ready, you do not have any advantage. You can train to get a tool out of your pocket or purse and get it ready, but it will take you at least a couple seconds to do so, even if you train about 50 hours the first year to do it. Remember, you will feel adrenaline, and the corresponding loss of coordination as well. After the first year, you will need to invest about 30 hours a year to maintain the same level of skill. Let's give you the benefit of the doubt and say you can get your tool out very quickly. For this example, let's use pepper spray. You have it in your pocket with nothing else, and you are able to just reach in and get it, twist it open, turn it the correct direction to aim it outwards, hold it steady, and now depress the trigger. Let's say you are amazingly fast and can do this in 1.5 seconds. Good so far? No, you're not.

Years ago, police officers were being killed more on the street, and they wanted to find out why. Studies showed that they were not getting their guns out in time. So they looked at how long it took to get the guns out and ready, and they said a well trained person could grip, unholster, raise, aim, and fire in not less than 1.5 seconds. Guess how far a motivated criminal can travel in 1.5 seconds? At an average of 14 feet per second, 21 feet. The 21 foot rule was born, and police have followed it ever since. That's why you see them draw their guns early and hold them at the low ready position now. They can't protect and serve you if they can't get their weapons out in time. Even if you have a concealed carry permit and carry a firearm, you should not attempt to draw and use it if the criminal is too close unless you have specific training for this, or it will not work for you.

So here's the reality. You have to train to get any Self Defense tool into position in just 1.5 seconds, and that takes a lot of practice. If someone is closer than 21 feet to you, you cannot bring your tool into position in time to use it. Since most criminal attacks are unexpected, Self Defense tools really create a false sense of security.

A lot of people reading this are probably very upset right now, and wondering what they should do. You should learn real Self Defense, and stop relying on a tool. There's nothing wrong with owning a tool, just understand the limitations of them, and don't rely on them for the immediate Self Defense need. If you are preparing for a transition, you can get your tool ready ahead of time. Just remember that with any tool, it can be taken from you and used against you if you do not know well how to use it or you are outnumbered as you would be in most criminal assaults.

Tactical Flashlights

The idea of a tactical flashlight is simple. An incredibly bright light spoils night vision, allowing you to create an opening. You can use this opening if you are law enforcement or military to ready a weapon, or if you are a civilian, you can use it to run to safety! Getting a tactical flashlight flashed in your eyes is startling and painful. What does it take to make a flashlight a 'tactical' flashlight? 300 lumens.

When these first came out, a student in my Martial Arts class brought one in. It was not commonly available yet, and was so expensive it was silly (more than $300), and was only used by law enforcement (he was SWAT). However, this light was something else, and made a big impression on me. This small handheld light was brighter than the 5 and 6 D battery mag lights that law enforcement had previously carried.

This was more than 20 years ago now, and times have changed. I just did a quick search on Amazon, and I found MANY tacticals for more than 300 lumens priced lower than $20. Originally these required very special and expensive batteries, and many still do, though if you prefer you can now find them with regular batteries, but they won't be as bright. If you get a flashlight like this, you will have to look carefully to make sure it includes a battery or that you buy the correct one separately. They are far from universal yet. Please keep this in mind.

Do you understand how night vision works? Your eyes have two parts that we are concerned with, rods and cones. During the day, you look right at something to see it clearly, which uses the cones. If it is dark and you look right at something, you actually won't see it that well. That's because cones are not designed to see well at night. For that, you need the rods. Rods work when you look out of the corner of your eye. That's why you can hear a funny noise at night and look right at it and never see it, then a critter scurries across your field of vision and you can see it from the corner of your eye, but again not when you look directly at it.

If it is dark out, and you are in a secure position, close your eyes for a few seconds. It helps your vision adapt much faster. When you open your eyes, if it is quite dark, remember not to look directly at things you want to see.

Your hands are powerful Self Defense tools. I like to keep mine empty and available. However, another strategy is to carry a tactical flashlight. If you do, you should put it in your non-dominant hand, so you are still able to use your dominant hand for Self Defense. If they put hands on you, drop the flashlight and use both hands as you resist. Your opportunity to use the flashlight has passed if they are already touching you.

Most tactical flashlights have a button with a couple different stages. Their default is off, then you press lightly and they will come on, release and they will turn off. Press harder and it will lock in the on position. I advocate that if you see or think you see something, flash the light there. If it is nothing to be concerned about, continue on. However, if it is a person sneaking in the dark or anything like that, flash it in their eyes and run the other way. You will want to practice so you just touch it on and off, that works far better for most Self Defense than it being continuously on. A flash and then gone takes a few seconds for your eyes to adjust, whereas you will more easily adjust to always on. Actually, some of these new lights are SO bright, brighter than I have used, so always on may now be a good option.

I'm overdue for a new light to play with. I'll update the www.immediateselfdefense.com recommendations page with info on a new light after I've had a chance to test them a bit.

Pepper Spray

The first thing you need to know about pepper spray is this: what are your local laws and ordinances regarding using it for Self Defense? Different places have different rules, and it's important to follow them. These days you hear a lot of people say that they will do whatever it takes, damn the rules, and then pay the consequences later; at least you are alive. I totally get this on one level, but we live in the real world here, so let's look at real situations.

Do you know that criminals frequently know the criminal justice system better than average citizens? It stands to reason, they spend more time around the system. Outside of jury duty and perhaps a speeding ticket, probably many people reading this have not even been into a court room. A repeat offending criminal has way more experience than you. They know loopholes and procedures, and they know how things work. They know the power of lying, and they will use it to make you look bad. "For no reason, this person just attacked me and shot me in the face with that stuff! I just asked them what time it was because I didn't have a watch!"

What this means is that if you have illegal pepper spray and use it on a criminal, they may well turn around and sue you. If they attack you and you beat them up in retaliation really really bad, they may sue you. It's kind of crazy, right? But it happens every day.

You need to know what pepper spray can do before you use it. It takes several steps to use pepper spray, so you would have to practice extensively: get it out of wherever it is and into your hand, remove the safety mechanism that prevents it from going off unintentionally, aim (nozzle at them, away from you), spray. Doing all those steps under pressure is a lot harder than you'd think, so you would need to practice them like any skill.

There are a lot of different kinds of pepper spray, and it does not affect people the same way. Also, pepper spray loses effectiveness, so you need to replace it every couple of years (regardless of what the packaging says). You need to find out what the legal limit on strength of pepper spray in your locality is before you buy it. In the USA, it seems to be regulated state by state. Something that is perfectly legal in one state will be highly illegal in another.

I've also seen some people advocating for carrying wasp spray and other things like this for Self Defense. Really? That stuff is big and awkward. Doesn't it seem too much? Plus, if it comes to court, how are you going to explain that you are carrying a huge bottle of something like that? If a criminal lies and says you started it, you can look bad because you were doing something ridiculous.

Mace vs Pepper Spray

A lot of people think these are really the same products. It's important to know that mace is a type of tear gas, and is not as commonly used today. It was thought to be not always as effective against people under the influence of alcohol and drugs as pepper spray. Some states prohibit the sale or use of mace by civilians. To add confusion to the situation, there is a popular brand of pepper spray called "Mace." I have not used Mace, and cannot speak to its effectiveness. However, pepper spray can be very effective, and if you get it in the eyes and mouth, it can work for up to 30 minutes. Pepper spray is also effective for dog and bear attacks. These days there are three dispersement types: spray, fogger, and gel. Spray aims well and shoots far, fogger creates a barrier that is perfect for multiple attackers, and gel will cause the criminal to wipe it away which will only make it worse. The added benefit of gel is that it is localized and will not enter the air, where you might breathe it too.

Careful

Ready for some craziness? Here in California, you can get a misdemeanor and even a Felony if you "display pepper spray in a threatening manner.". It is best used for Self Defense without advertising that you are going to use it.

Tasers

I don't like them. I don't think they are reasonable for most people. You face the same problems of needing to have them with you, needing to have them accessible, and needing to have time to bring them to bear. Only people HIGHLY trained should use them. The worst thing about them is that they are not appropriate for a huge number of situations, and that requires the kind of thought that you don't have time to make unless you have LOTS of experience. If you are law enforcement and you are going to carry them, make sure you get lots of training. If you are doing training, it is NOT recommended and in fact highly discouraged for you to be tased multiple times. Doing so, according to even the taser manufacturers and not just the complainants, can "impair breathing and respiration."

If you are a civilian, I highly discourage you from having a taser. There are a lot of regulations around ownership, possession, and use of tasers, so please find out what restrictions your area has before you buy one. You are not limited to national and state or province regulations, but there may be local regulations too. (For instance, they cannot be carried by anyone but law enforcement for any reason on the college campus I teach at). In the right circumstances they are SO effective that they can easily give you a totally false sense of confidence, and you might not get the training that you need for all the other circumstances.) Remember that most person-to-person crimes are not usually committed by a lone criminal, but in pairs or threes. You will only be able to control one of them with the taser at best.

There are essentially two types of tasers. One shoots electrodes that stay in your skin by darts on wires fired by nitrogen. If they make a halfway decent connection, they will drop anyone. They must be used within very specific range, and with all but the most expensive models you have just one shot. They are working to improve the technology, and there is a lot of promise on the horizon, but the most expensive models still have just 3 shots currently.

The second type of taser is called a "drive stun" or "stun gun." Drive stun is where you depress the switch or turn it on, and press the electrodes against the skin. Some of these newer drive stun devices can reach deeper and so are still very effective against a layer of clothes.

There are, of course, hybrids which allow both the true taser on electrode and the drive stun. These models are common for law enforcement. Drive stun can be done without the air cartridge, or after the taser has already been used and the air cartridge has deployed.

Each time a taser is deployed, it shoots out confetti with the serial numbers on them. This is collected at a scene, along with the cartridge, and booked into evidence to document whose taser was used and how many times. The officer should also take pictures of the puncture sites and call for medical attention. Some tasers for law enforcement now have cameras built into them. Each deployment is documented in a police report, as well as any verbal warnings before the taser was used.

A Few More Notes on Tasers

Tasers should never be aimed at the eyes or face. If you have a taser, you must clearly understand the safety feature. Tasers cannot be carried on board an aircraft – they must be in checked luggage. Before you travel with a taser, check the laws in the areas you are traveling to and from. There are expiration dates on the air cartridges, and they must be kept current. Tasers are not as effective at very close range, and are ineffective at over 15 feet. Tasers are designed to be used from 20 degrees to 115 degrees, and may not function outside this range. The inside of your car will get too hot for a taser.

Impact Training

Impact training is an important part of your arsenal. Impact training is any kind of strike to a target, whether it be a heavy bag, hand pad, or to a person wearing protective gear. The ability to deliver impact is very important, and must be trained. An untrained person is highly ineffective in this area. A trained person is instantly dangerous and cannot be disarmed or have their weapons taken away and used against them. It is not as difficult to be trained as you might think; it just requires qualified instruction.

There are several factors that can make you far more effective instantly, but they are easy to misunderstand. If you do them wrong, you lose a lot of potential impact. You have to learn to use your body in a coordinated way. Stepping to put your whole mass into motion, pushing from the ground, pivoting your hips, using your shoulders, all the muscles, bones, and joints doing the right motions the right way at the right timing, and bang, you are incredibly effective. If you add recoil and retraction, you are two or three times more effective (otherwise you are just pushing, and not delivering impact). Proper impact almost makes the attacker feel like you were in a car accident. It's shocking how much force even a very small person can deliver, especially when they use the right targets (covered in another section).

When you are training impact, you have to approach the subject from a lot of different viewpoints. You have to work in a static way, in place, learning to connect your body to a target in front of you in various ways. You have to work on turning to different angles by stepping forward, back, and turning and delivering impact. You have to work on being surprised and having to deliver impact. You have to work on breaking free from various holds and delivering impact. There's a lot to work on. You'll find, however, that you are naturally much better than you expect you are. We humans have very good instincts; I just think they are a little buried by modern society. You can wake them back up with relative ease, and be more effective than ever. Once you wake them up, they are easy to maintain.

The thing that you have to realize most about impact training is that it is never perfect. You must, however, continue to work on it and it will get much much better. If your progress ever stagnates, you need another way to work on the skill, because progress has no limit when it comes to this kind of training.

The flip side of impact training is receiving impact. If you really want to be good, you need to feel what it is like to be hit. Now stay with me. I know a bunch of you are about to put the book down and never pick it up again. What you'll discover is that your body is actually very resilient. You can take a lot more than you think and keep on fighting. This is why it's so important to fight back. A criminal is only fighting for their dinner; if you are a hard target, they'll go somewhere else. You, however, are fighting for your life. You can put everything you have into surviving, and you will do it. It is far more a mindset than it is a physical skill. There are very safe ways to work on receiving impact. Make sure if you are learning this, you are learning from someone qualified. (They are not just beating you up, there are methods of training so you can learn all the specific skills required.)

Static training is best done on a heavy bag. Not too heavy, mind you, because the body will move when you hit it. You don't want a bag so heavy that it only stays in place no matter what, as that leads to unrealistic training. Nothing over 100 pounds is really useful because of this fact. There are lots of great brands. If you are training regularly, ask your teacher what they like. Shipping can be a huge factor; they may have a local supplier.

If you are doing a lot of impact training, it can wear on your hands. You will want to buy "Bag Balm" in the green can. You can find it lots of places. If you don't see it near you, it is on Amazon. It will help your hands heal much faster.

I have these recommendations and a discussion of their benefits on my website: http://immediateselfdefense.com/recommendations

Weapons Training

I love weapons training. It might be my favorite. I don't feel that I can really do weapons training any justice in a book. The subject is advanced, and requires seeing, feeling, and doing in person. In addition to training with everyday weapons like knives and sticks and weapons of opportunity, I train with many weapons from Japan, Okinawa, and China. If you are interested in training with weapons, we frequently do trainings of all different kinds. If you are learning a weapon, it is important to really hit, poke, and/or cut with it. There are safe ways to do this. Come join us or host me for a special event at your location. Let's talk. Weapons training can revolutionize and reinvigorate your practice. Stick and knife training is part of our weekend intensive trainings.

Clothing & Gear

Clothing and training gear is very individual. Here is some advice I can give you. In the Martial Arts, we usually wear uniforms, because our training is hard on our regular clothes. In fact, in Okinawa, it was common practice to take off their clothes and practice in their underwear so as not to ruin their clothes. Everyone was very happy when the founder of Judo, Jigoro Kano, introduced the uniform, modeled after traditional style clothing, and made it strong enough to last. It was quickly adopted into Karate and the other arts in Okinawa.

Even if you like training in a uniform like I do (saves on the clothing bills), you should, from time to time, wear regular clothes (just not your newest, fanciest, favorite stuff, because it WILL get ruined). The great thing about a uniform is that it is unrestrictive, so you can learn well, and there are some very durable brands, that will hold up to vigorous use. In contrast, it is important to train sometimes in regular clothes, because you must know if and how much your clothing restricts your movements, and feel how it will give way or change things in real movement.

This consideration is especially important for shoes. Gentlemen, many dressy shoes have fairly slick bottoms. If you are going to wear them, you need to have some practice in them in Self Defense situations so you understand how they can affect your leverage. (I personally only wear dressy shoes with some tread.) Ladies, if you like to wear high heeled shoes, you should have some time practicing Self Defense while wearing them so you know what adjustments you need to make. (A heel on a foot can be very effective.)

When you are training, you will want to make sure that your clothing is comfortable for you, even when you are sweating, and especially as you are moving around vigorously. Just try putting your clothes through a workout and you'll see how they do. For training shoes, my very favorite are Adidas Samba, a type of indoor soccer shoe with a wide base and a series of concentric circles at the ball of the foot called a turning point. These shoes allow me to turn comfortably without undue wear and tear. You can use any shoes you like or none, depending on your environment (I frequently train barefoot), but training can take a wear and tear on your shoe. Getting the right shoes will save you money, and wear and tear on your feet, ankles, and knees. You should periodically practice with any shoes that you frequently wear, so you see how they do.

Whatever you do, don't let not having the ideal equipment and gear stop you from training. It's well worth your time to get training from the right source, and to work on whatever exercises you are given on your own or with good training partners. Equipment is secondary. Mindset is the most important.

Chapter 9
Special Considerations

What If You Are Assaulted?

During the assault, the most important consideration is to fight back and never give up. Look for an opportunity to break free and run. These should be the only thoughts in your head, your only considerations. If you make it hard enough, the criminal will give up and find another target instead. All experts agree that fighting back is your best strategy.

After the Assault

If you have been assaulted, I hope that you were able to run away and that you are safe. Regardless of what happened, if you are alive to tell about it, you are far luckier than some. It might be hard to be grateful right about now, but you are lucky to be alive.

You will want to make sure to call emergency services (the police), and get help. If there is any evidence to gather or photos to take, you want them to have this opportunity. The sooner the better after the assault, when the evidence is fresh. Another section of this chapter discusses how to conduct yourself with 9-1-1 or emergency services, and another talks about how to give descriptions of persons and vehicles for police reports. Filing a police report is critical. Most criminals are repeat offenders, and the reason it takes so long to finally get them off the streets, is that people don't follow through and do the reports, bring charges with a lawyer, follow up in court, etc.

If you have visible marks on your body, the police will likely take all photos necessary, but if you are not sure, have someone you trust take more. You want to document anything visible after an assault. And again after a couple days if new bruising or injuries are now surfacing.

You need to seek medical attention. Get checked by a professional. Make sure you are really ok. You need to put taking care of yourself first. Some people feel very vulnerable right after an assault, and some are more in shock, and do not seem to process what has happened for a time. You should consider counseling. It has helped many people in similar situations.

To add insult to injury, if your wallet and personal information was stolen, the criminal may try to steal your identity, or sell your information to someone else who will do so. There is a section in this chapter addressing this.

Do not be alone for a while. If at all possible, be around people you trust. Criminals often repeat offend against the same victims. You will not only feel safer around people, you will actually BE safer.

Most importantly, know that you are not at fault. The victim is never at fault. The criminal is. It doesn't matter if you know them or not, you are not responsible in any way for the attack; all the blame belongs to the criminal.

It is common, after an assault, for your emotions to be running high for quite some time. You may not feel like you are stressed, but you may find that small things that never would have bothered you before are now very stressful or even overwhelming. This is very normal. The easiest way to get through this time is to have a regular exercise routine. If you do not have a trainer, consider getting one, so you have someone to hold you accountable (a workout buddy may work too, but they need to be very reliable). Exercise is a very natural and healthy way to reduce all kinds of stress and give yourself an outlet. If you have access to a heavy bag and someone to teach you how, learn how to hit the heavy bag. It is excellent therapy. At all costs, avoid sitting around thinking about the assault over and over and trying to figure out what you did "wrong." Remember, it is not your fault. Take care of yourself first.

Vehicle Strategies

I like to work on things that other Self Defense teachers might find unusual. I have heard about all different sorts of scenarios where people were assaulted, and I like to put myself in those situations and work on solutions to these problems using the basic principles we already know. What I've found, without exception, is that the principles we teach work well in all environments, you just have to also account for the environment and different opportunities or limitations they provide.

As a result, I teach a lot of different concepts of Self Defense from a car. Being inside a car severely limits your mobility, so it is surprisingly common how often criminals will use the car as a way to create an opening.

Let's start from if you are driving a car. If you are driving down the road with your windows down and come to a stop, a criminal can suddenly run out, reach inside your vehicle, and put a gun to your chest/face/head to take the car. If this happens, give up the car and run. Your life is worth more than a car. (This actually happened several times in my town one year recently.) The problem could have been avoided by having the window rolled up. The criminals did not approach anyone with the window up, because they could not reach inside.

Another common tactic criminals use, if you are already driving, is to put something in the road that you will run over and that will make a lot of noise or cause you to have to stop. When you stop, they are waiting for you. I am not saying if you run over something and you want to stop that you should not, but I am saying that you need to have your wits about you. If something doesn't feel right, it probably isn't. Don't instantly turn off your vehicle. If people are rapidly approaching your vehicle and you get a bad feeling or see weapons, drive quickly and get out of there. Cars will drive through most anything if they are not badly damaged. Having AAA or some type of roadside assistance is a good idea in these situations too.

If you have been away from your car, before you get back into it, walk around the car and check it. First look to see if anyone is watching you. They may be trying to see if you have a lapse in awareness and you are vulnerable. Then look inside the car (make sure someone is not hiding in the back seat), then look at the tires (make sure they are all inflated). It is very common for criminals to assault you at your car. If everything is ok, don't just get into your car and hang out there for a long time checking your makeup or your email. If you are not in a public, well-lighted place, you should get into your car and drive. Criminals love a person who is not paying attention and is a sitting duck. If you are inside your car and you see someone unknown approaching your car, lock the doors, roll up the window, turn on the car, and leave. Even if they are just asking for spare change, it is a common strategy for criminals to work together. One will "spare change" you and pull your attention one direction, while another will slip into your car if it is unlocked, and assault you.

In my intensive weekend trainings, I teach several techniques from inside the car. We have techniques for when you are sitting in the driver's seat and the attacker is outside, for sitting in the passenger seat and the attacker is outside, for sitting in the passenger seat and attacked from the back seat, for sitting in the driver seat and attacked from the back seat, from two attackers, what if they have weapons, and more. The concepts are not really very different, but it is important to practice with having the steering wheel and pedals in your way and not.

Lastly, we cover what to do it you are outside a car and assaulted. A car can be a powerful weapon for you, even if it is parked. You just have to know how to use it.

Defensive Driving

You might be an amazing driver, but another driver might not be, or might be drunk. I have had good results with avoiding accidents by following these rules of defensive driving:

- Always leave plenty of time to get from one place to another
- Plan your route in advance
- Leave plenty of room between your car and the next car
- Use your mirrors and look over your shoulder. Other drivers may not see you
- Give bicyclists plenty of room
- When in doubt, wait for the right opportunity
- Use your turn signals
- Watch for changing conditions
- Consider the weather
- Be alert and avoid distractions (avoid music being too loud, cellphone use, etc.)
- Expect other drivers to make mistakes, and be prepared to react

Stolen Wallet/Phone, Identity Theft

- Have a backup of all information
- Have a list of phone numbers of banks and credit cards
- Call credit cards and banks, explain the situation, request new account numbers
- If you have lost checks, close your account and open a new one. To prevent yourself from facing the costs if a criminal uses your

checks at a merchant's cash register, the FTC recommends calling these check verification services:

Certegy (800) 77-3792

TeleCheck (800) 710-9898

International Check Services (800) 631-9656

- Open a police report for your stolen wallet or purse
- Call credit agencies and request a fraud alert
  Experian – 1-888-EXPERIAN
  Equifax – 1-800-525-6285
  Trans Union – 1-800-680-7289
- Start watching your credit report www.annualcreditreport.com. This is the free annual credit report that everyone is entitled to by law
- Report your driver's license stolen to police and DMV. To get a duplicate driver's license, you will have to go in person to the DMV with one or two forms of ID, like passport, social security, or birth certificate
- If your social security number is abused, file a complaint with the Federal Trade Commission. www.ftccomplaintassistant.gov or call 1-877-438-4338
- If your keys are stolen, change the locks on your home and car. Even if your keys are recovered, criminals could have copied the keys
- Consider a service like Lifelock. I have not used one, but I know people who were living a nightmare, and Lifelock was able to help.

If your identity is stolen, you need to be vigilant about defending it for at least two years.

Smartphone

As soon as you get a new smartphone, put a password on it and change it regularly. There are now many kinds of apps that will set off an alarm, track the phone, lock the phone, and even remote wipe (erase data) from the phone. Make sure to regularly do backups of any information you need (to cloud or a desktop computer). Know your serial number (keep it someplace safe when you first get your phone). Your service provider may also have your serial number.

If your phone is lost or stolen, report it to the police (making sure to tell them about the security app you have installed), and report it to the service provider so they can stop any new charges to your account or credit card. Police may ask for the serial number.

If you have an iPhone, you can sign in to icloud.com/find on any computer, or use the Find My Phone app on another iDevice. Turn on Lost Mode. This will stop the phone from being able to use Apple Pay with your credit or debit cards. You can even keep track of your device's location. If you erase your iDevice, you can no longer track it. If you remove it from your account after you erase it, activation lock is turned off. A criminal can then activate and use your device.

Authorities: Emergency Services, Police Descriptions of Persons and Vehicles

Calling 9-1-1 or your local number for Emergency Services
Do not hang up and redial – you will only delay a response.

Listen carefully to their questions, answer all their questions well but briefly – this is not the time for a long story. They are trying to sort out exactly what kind of help you need and who is best to send. Be clear, be brief, listen.

They dispatch by priority – anything that is an immediate threat to life, injury, or major property damage is higher.

Use the non-emergency number when an immediate personal response is not necessary

Examples of what they may ask you

- what is your emergency
- what is your location and cross-street
- if you saw something, what did you see (be brief)
- is anyone hurt (triggers them to call emergency medical services and/or fire department)
- if you witnessed a crime and you saw someone fleeing, they will ask which direction and for a description (more info below)
- is anyone still a threat on scene
- your name and info, stay on the line

Police descriptions – Person

If you see a suspicious person, or have an encounter you need to report, here is what the police will want to know when you give a description:

- Gender
- Race
- Age
- Height/Weight
- Color Hair/Eyes
- Clothing
- Unusual characteristics: glasses, beard, jewelry, visible tattoos
- Location last seen
- Direction of travel

Police descriptions – Vehicle

If you need to report a vehicle to the police, here is the information they will ask you for:

- 2 or 4 door, van, pickup, or SUV
- make of vehicle
- color
- license number & state
- number of people in the vehicle & describe the people

- unusual characteristics of the vehicle: dents, marks, stickers
- location last seen
- direction of travel

When Help Arrives

If you have someone who can wait in a visible place for help to arrive, then do so. They should wave or "flag down" emergency responders, and direct them to where they need to go. Listen carefully and answer briefly to any questions they may ask you. Do not guess what info they need; just listen carefully, and briefly give them the info they ask for only.

If you are a victim or you witnessed a crime, the responding officer will ask you what happened. They will want to know if you are the only eyewitness, or if others were there. If there are other witnesses, the officer will talk to everyone. They will ask if you know the suspects. They will ask if you were to see the criminal, if you would be recognize them. If so, they will set up a photo lineup in the future. Regardless of whether you are the victim or the reporting party, they will get your info, address, driver's license number, phone, etc. They will ask you what/why/and what time. If you need medical attention, the officer may go with you to the hospital to find out the extent of the injuries. This determines the charges that may be filed. If there is only minor bruising and you don't need to see a doctor, it may be only a misdemeanor. However, if you are unconscious or need to see a doctor, it may be a felony. The more serious the injury, the more serious the response. They may rope off the area for evident collection such as spent casings or cigarette butts, clothing, DNA from suspects.

The first responding officer will take a handwritten statement, and this report becomes the criminal investigation. The better job they are able to do with the help of witnesses, etc., the more info the police will have to go on to resolve the case. The investigating officer will try to determine why the crime occurred. Security cameras are a big help these days! Crime tip hotlines can also be a very important tool. The patrolman files the initial report, and the detectives will follow up. They file a criminal complaint with the District Attorney (D.A.). It is up to the D.A. to determine which cases to try, and which not to try. A lot goes into making a conviction. Every bit of info you have is useful.

Safety Net Workers

Let me take just this one moment to say thank you to all of our safety net workers. Thank you to all law enforcement, 911 operators, emergency medical services, firemen, support personnel, and military of all branches. It is because of your continued sacrifices that the rest of us get to enjoy our freedom and quality of life. I can't say thank you enough.

Whenever you interact with anyone in one of these tough jobs, please be respectful and make it easy for them to do their job. They have to see and deal with things that the rest of us get to live blissfully ignorant of. They have a tough job to do, and a lot of people truly don't appreciate their efforts for our benefit.

There is a tendency these days for people to be very untrusting of law enforcement. This is really unfortunate, because almost 100% of them get into the career because they really believe in helping people. If the public is defensive, disrespectful, and untrusting, it really makes their job much harder, and can put them at greater risk. Please be kind and respectful with law enforcement. It will make their difficult job easier. If there really is a problem with a specific officer, take it up the chain of command. The sergeant, lieutenant, and so on to the Chief will want to know if there is a problem so they can address it.

Medical Attention

If you are the victim of an assault, it is important to get checked out. If you are a victim of a sexual assault, be sure to get any medical testing done before taking a shower and losing valuable evidence. If you are a victim of a sexual assault, it is also important to get checked for STDs. Sometimes people don't because they don't want to know, but not knowing might increase your problems. Treatment, if any is needed, is best administered at the right time, not waiting until it is an emergency. I understand how awkward and awful just thinking about all of this may be. That's why it's ideal to learn this before anything happens, so that if, god forbid, something DOES happen, you know the right steps, you've already considered what to do and you make the good decision. Most sexual predators are repeat offenders. Evidence that you might be able to provide can help get that person off the streets, and help protect other people and even yourself (the unfortunate truth is that victims are often re-victimized by the same criminal if they do not report. You see, the criminal has found someone they think is an easy target, and criminals always go for what's easy).

If you are not certain if you need medical attention, it is still better to check. Have you even been in a car accident or had a concussion? You might feel like you are OK at the moment, but later that day, the next day, even two days later you might find it is a very different story.

Emotional, Psychological, and Philosophical Changes

People who suffer criminal assault frequently go through emotional, psychological, and philosophical changes. What I mean by this is that you might have been very naïve before, and believed that all people were good, because that had been your experience. Afterwards, you might have a hard time feeling this way. However, you should know, the vast majority of people ARE very good. You just need to be sure to be around them as much as possible, and learn how to stay away from the bad ones. Many victims of assault benefit from counseling. If you have been a victim, please consider it.

Photographing Evidence

Real life is not like what you see on TV or in the movies. Your clothes may be torn. You might very well have lots of cuts and scrapes. You might develop bruises after a day or two. All of these issues need to be documented with pictures and/or video, and possibly affidavits from witnesses. (I am not a lawyer; consult a lawyer for legal advice pertinent to where you live.) When you file a police report, they will probably take care of taking all the pictures you need. I recommend not only immediate photos, but also following up a couple days later. You may find that new marks have developed that were not obvious before. If you have professional help, perfect, please consult your professional and take their advice.

Do Not Be Alone

If you should suffer a criminal assault, take my advice. Don't be anywhere alone for a few days. Your emotions will be on edge, and you will react to every little sound, real or imagined. Humans are social creatures. You will do better with people around you. Take care of your safety and security – criminals often repeat offend on the same victim. Being alone puts you at greater risk; don't do it. Give yourself the space and time you need to heal. Everyone will understand. Take care of yourself first, above all.

Emotions and Trauma

Being the victim of an assault is not a fun experience. There are so many different kinds of reactions, and your process of healing may not be the same as someone else's. You may not even feel that you really experienced much trauma and may feel fine, but years later, the unresolved issue may come back up.

Trauma is a complex subject, and there is no one size fits all model. There is a great deal of debate in the field of traumatic stress on the value of talking it out and revisiting the traumatic memory. The problem is that some people find talking about it incredibly helpful, while others find it to be very damaging. When even the professionals don't agree, you know it is a complex topic, one that depends a lot on each person.

After a traumatic event, many people feel unsafe. You may not feel safe in your own skin, in your home, or in your relationships (if someone who had what should have been a safe, supporting relationship with you assaults you, this is especially true). Your first priority should be to get safe. Change your environment if necessary, so you feel that you can be safe. You need to create a stable environment for yourself.

You may experience extremely volatile emotions including denial, anger, numbness (almost no emotions), trouble sleeping, inability to concentrate, memory problems, etc. While many professionals understand and advocate for trauma survivors to do things like deep breathing exercises, yoga, and qigong, I find that very few professionals mention exercise. This is really a shame, because the easiest way to emotional mastery is through exercise. It's completely built into our physiology; it is part of flight or flight. When adrenaline and stress happens, and you fight or flee, you will automatically reset your body and recover well. However, if you freeze (the other common response, like a deer in headlights), you get no benefits, and your body stays agitated because you did not react.

If you ever are having wild emotions and need to control them and calm yourself down, the kind of exercise you need is vigorous, and it needs to be sustained for a period of time. 15 to 20 minutes is ideal. Your heart rate needs to go up, your pores need to open, and you need to sweat. AFTER this is the ideal time to do deep breathing, yoga, and qigong. This is the ideal way to get all the benefits.

I have an analogy that I think is helpful, so stay with me here. You are the water, your emotions are the knob that adjusts how hot the stove is, and the stove is your environment. Put water on a cold stove, and the water will not heat. Turn the stove up high, put the water on the stove, and it will heat up quickly! All that is changed here is the temperature setting (your emotions). You may not be able to control your environment (sometimes we can, sometimes we can't). What you CAN control is your temperature setting (your emotions), but that takes some doing. If what someone else can say or do affects your emotions, you have given them control. You put the knob in their hand and let them adjust your stove. Take the power back! Become the one who keeps control of their own temperature setting.

This is a lot easier to say than it is to do. No one is perfect, and you will certainly lose your cool. When you realize you have lost it, collect yourself, maybe even remove yourself from the environment (take the water off the stove for a bit), and get control again.

The best way we have of regulating our emotions is vigorous exercise. Emotional regulation is in fact the most powerful reason to exercise, not weight loss (weight loss requires careful attention to what you eat, like saving money takes careful attention to what you spend and where you could cut back on wasteful spending). When you build a habit of exercise, it can be a very powerful benefit in your life. When your emotions are well regulated, you will be your best self. You will be calm, so you will be more kind and patient. You will not overreact to circumstances around you; instead you will see things from a different perspective.

If this section was meaningful for you, more of these "internal" topics will be found in a future book on lessons of leadership learned through the study of Martial Arts. You can also visit my website, www.leaderlessons.com.

Chapter 10
Ongoing Learning

What is your goal?

What is your goal for ongoing learning? When you begin with the end in mind, you are already halfway there, because you won't have to retrace your steps and start over. Determining your goal is an important first step. Get clear about your goals in learning, then you can know who and what kind of class/teacher can help you to achieve your goal.

This then begs the question, which kinds of goals are there? And how do I choose a goal? Let me help. Your first determination must be, do you want to learn Self Defense or Martial Arts? They are not the same, as we have discussed at length in this book. The next chapter will discuss what to look for in a Self Defense course, and the chapter after that, what to look for in a Martial Arts class. But how do you choose? Simple. How much time are you willing to devote to your training? If you are not willing to devote a minimum of 2-3 hours per week for several years, you should not study Martial Arts. With less time and attention than that, you will get very little out of it compared to what you could, and worse still, you will not get enough hands-on Self Defense as part of your other training to make it truly worthwhile from a Self Defense perspective. Martial Arts are designed to be studied for your whole life; the black belt has been widely misunderstood to mean expert, when it truly means you have passed the pre-requisites, and are now ready for advanced study.

If your goal is fitness, and thereby an increased ability to run away or fight back in case of danger (a worthy goal), then you need the right kind of training. Full body workouts would be ideal. Be sure to mix cardio and weight training or some form of resistance training into your routine. Being part of a class would allow you to have a social group, which can help you keep on track. If you have the extra money, having a personal trainer is highly desirable because they can help you to do things correctly. Also, simply having an appointment that you are paying for will force you to be more consistent, which leads to much better results. The ideal is to have a social group to work out together with, and supplement this with personal training instruction.

If your desire is Self Defense, you should find several people near you that teach this, and go watch some classes, or participate in low cost trainings and don't sign any contracts for more money until you know that you want to learn from them. You may also consider my website, www.immediateselfdefense.com, or in-person training with me.

If your desire is Martial Arts, you should find several different Martial Arts schools and go watch their classes. You will want to watch the instructors and the students, see if you want to learn there, from them, in the way that they teach, and if you want to get the results that the students have gotten. You may also consider my video training, available through my website, www.martialarts academy.online or in-person training with me (Self Defense is the basis of everything that I do, but I teach several different Martial Arts, armed and unarmed, in the traditional way).

In addition to your desired goal, you must also consider yourself. Do you have any physical limitations that would prohibit you from doing certain things? If this is the case, you need to find someone who understands that limitation, so that you can get the most out of your training. At the very least, you must work with someone who can appreciate your limitation, and find creative ways to work with you to allow you to do all that you can do. You may find that with some training, some limitations lesson or even go away (some will certainly not).

What to look for in a Self Defense Course

As we discussed already, the needs of students of a Self Defense course and a Martial Arts class are fundamentally different. Here are a few things that are crucial for Self Defense. Techniques must be clear and simple. The more complicated, the less chance that you will be able to access those skills under pressure because of adrenaline. Techniques must work well for people of all sizes; they cannot be dependent on size or strength, but instead must work with your whole body in a coordinated way.

If you are doing a technique that requires you to grip in exactly a certain way at exactly a certain point, you are going to fail, unless you invest hundreds if not thousands of hours on that skill under pressure. In real life, people move quite a bit, and things happen very quickly. Simple concepts work much better.

Mobility vs. Stability is an important consideration for Self Defense. If what you are learning requires you to have your feet on the ground in a stable way, you are in serious danger. It's counterintuitive, isn't it? Wouldn't stability be good? Yes, it certainly can be, however, the problem is, that if you are stable, you are planting your weight, and dedicated to holding your ground. Now all you need is someone bigger and stronger, or two people smaller than you, and they will easily control your body because you are actively resisting by trying to hold your ground. It is FAR more effective, instead, to learn to move. As much as possible, whatever you learn, should work without requiring you to hold your ground. If you can move in, move out, circle, and still use the technique, then you are at less risk of falling down or being taken to the ground. Now if you love Martial Arts ground techniques, cool, so do I. However, the problem with them for Self Defense is that you NEVER know that you have just one attacker. You could easily start with one, and then another joins. If you are on the ground against two people, you are in serious trouble. There are things you can do still, but if you can avoid this situation, you absolutely should. In real life, you are not inside a cage like you see on TV where no one else can get to you and you have a one-on-one fight. You will never know how many people might be involved until after it is all over.

I teach a lot of drills to address mobility and stability. We learn how to keep ourselves in the ideal posture to both resist force, and to use force. We learn how to keep our leverage good and make use of our mechanical advantage, while always compromising the criminal's leverage and position. The reflexes you need are already part of your nervous system; you just need to wake them up. We work a lot on footwork, because with improper footwork, you might get taken to the ground, which we want to avoid if at all possible as we already discussed.

A good course should address not just single person attacks from the front, but from all sides. The course should address ambushes, blind spots, how night vision works (if it is pitch black and you look right at something, you will not see it, you need instead to look out of the corner of your eye using the rods instead of the cones, which see well during the day and directly in front of you, but not well at all in darkness). The course should address common strategies that criminals use, such as distraction, misdirection, and confusion. It should address various kinds of approaches, such as single front, front and side, front and rear, etc. It should address various kinds of grabbing assaults and holds, but these should be simply presented, and there should be no complicated memorization.

Everything you learn should not be dependent on being able to see, because it might be dark or you might otherwise have bad visibility (something covering the face is often used in abductions).

Everything should be based on feel and response to pressure instead. The biggest physical factor is that it should not rely on strength, speed, or any other physical attribute (though the more fit and strong you are, the easier everything will work), but instead, what you learn should be based on applying your entire mass to small leverage points so that it works quite easily. (An example is that if someone is grabbing you with both hands, wrap your arms around their elbow and drop your weight down and spring back up. This puts all your leverage on one small joint, which will make their grip fail. You are bigger than their arm. Concepts like this are best experienced in person, though you may also see examples of these principles on my website, www.immediateselfdefense.com.)

What to Look for in a Martial Arts Class

Everyone is different, and likely everyone will want to get something different out of their Martial Arts class. I could get very specific about different styles, lineages, etc., but that would be based on my preferences and knowledge, and might not apply perfectly to your circumstance. Instead, I'm going to be very general about certain things, but very specific about others.

There are LOTS of different styles out there. But I'm going to say something that will probably shock many other martial artists, and they very well may not agree. As much as I love the styles I have learned, I don't think most students should pay much attention to style. Thinking that one style is better than one another is very simplistic. Maybe my opinion is different because I've been lucky enough to learn and teach several styles at a very high level, and I've been even MORE lucky to visit with and work with teachers from many other styles. I truly think that every style that I have tried was really great.

Each style has specific things that they tend to emphasize, and others that they de-emphasize, at least in the beginning. However, that often changes as you make your way through the ranks and curriculum, so many styles end up offering a very well-rounded curriculum. Even if your teacher does not know something that you are interested in, that does not mean that they cannot get you that knowledge and skill. A teacher often has access to and relationships with many other teachers. A great teacher will see that you have certain natural abilities and/or interests, and if these are somewhat different than their own, they will help you build a relationship with another teacher. With your teacher's blessing and introduction, the second teacher may well tell you and show you things that otherwise you would never see, or put you on a fast track to learning and gaining those skills. Every great teacher loves having a great student, so referring your best students to other teachers is a common way that teachers build friendships between them, with students that are very sincere and trustworthy. I have benefitted from this tremendously, the same way that my teacher did before me. Because he was a wonderful student, his teachers and mentors went out of their way to give him opportunities that he would otherwise never have had. In turn my teacher did that for me, and the teachers and mentors that he introduced me to have also done this for me. It's really a win win for everyone. I do the same for my own students, now it's my turn to pay it forward.

The real question about any style is, is it interesting to you? Is it what you are interested in studying? By spending your time, will you gain the skills and knowledge that you are looking for? Are you able to learn well and effectively from the teacher you are studying with? Are you doing both general classes and private lessons for more detailed and personalized instruction? That's certainly a fast track to better and better skills. Doing private lessons will allow you to learn and improve without so many of the common missteps that practice with less direction can accidentally create. In some ways, the more you invest financially, the more committed you will be, and the more you will focus on your goals.

When you watch a class, are the students and not only the instructor exhibiting the skillsets that you would like to have? Something to realize is, that you will only gain these skills if you consistently and persistently practice, both at the lessons and away on your own. If it is not interesting to you, you will have a hard time being consistent. Even so, a great way to keep your motivation going is to make friends with the other students and bring your friends to also become students of the Martial Arts school.

Online Learning

It is much better to learn in person. Certain skills would be difficult if not impossible to really understand without hands-on training in person. You may, however, be in a place where you do not have access regular access in person to the teacher or style that you would like to learn. It is also possible that you have a work schedule or personal circumstance that does not allow you to regularly learn in person. If that is your circumstance, then please do not just go to google or youtube and start trying to watch everything and anything in an attempt to learn.

If regular learning in person is not possible, you would still get some benefit from following an online training program, especially if there is a way for you to at least work in person with that instructor sometimes for key points. Without a personal relationship with the instructor and other students, it is also easy to get lost or lose your initial spark of interest, so in person learning is far preferable. The truth is, certain things you will not be able to understand without hands-on instruction period.

www.immediateselfdefense.com

My website for Self Defense has some FREE videos that are accessible to everyone, a members area for a monthly cost (discount for yearly), and corporate discounts for multiple memberships. With corporate membership, you can also use the PDF notes in your own print publications, and the videos in your own electronic publications.

www.martialartsacademy.online

I also have a website devoted to the 501c3 non-profit Martial Arts school I founded, Martial Arts Academy Bujutsu Gakuin Wushu Xueyuan. I teach Okinawan Karate, both Matsubayashi Shorin Ryu and Goju Ryu, and many classical Okinawan weapons from several traditions. I teach Japanese Swordsmanship: Iaido, Kenjutsu, Kendo, and Batto Do. My base is Muso Jikiden Eishin Ryu. I teach some Arnis de Mano, a stick fighting system from the Philippines that is really fun to learn and practice. I teach Yang Style Taijiquan and Qigong. I emphasize the functional aspects of Taijiquan (Tai Chi) training, and the health benefits of Qigong (Chi Kung). Finally, I teach 7 Star Praying Mantis Kung Fu, a highly complex system that takes more than dedication to master. The thing I like best about what I've learned is that I never just learned forms, I always focused on function and the why and how of everything. I've been fortunate to have an amazing teacher, Tim McFarland, both a Sensei and a Shifu (Sifu) guide me all along the way, and provide me opportunities to work with and learn from so many amazing teachers, too many to mention. Through him and his friends, training opportunities have come that have been truly amazing.

Other Styles

Many of the major styles have a variety of websites available, and you may find some distance learning programs out there. As with anything, caveat emptor, let the buyer beware. Before you pay much, make sure it is something you are really interested in, and that learning in that way works for you. Remember that without a personal relationship with a teacher, they cannot refer you to other experts. You won't gain access to the very best Martial Arts skills just by asking, you have to have an introduction to the right people. Martial Arts are no different than anything else in that way; who you know matters a lot.

Seminars for Hands-On Learning

As I've discussed, there is simply no substitute for hands-on learning. Many of the people who might prefer to train with me do not live close to me. I do travel and teach groups, individuals, and corporations, and you may also consider traveling to learn. I like to do brief introductions for people just getting exposure or reviewing (2 to 5 hours), because I believe everyone should learn Self Defense. These tend to be very affordable, especially when you consider the value of the learning and training. Consider for a moment, what the value of hands-on learning would be. It could be life-changing. You might learn something well that could literally save the life of yourself or a loved one. Frankly I could probably charge almost any amount, and it would be worth it. However, I want to reach lots and lots of people and put the information and knowledge in their hands, so I make at least the basic training very affordable and accessible. If you are interested in scheduling something in your area, reach out to me, and let's see what we can work out. My contact information is included here in the book, or reach me through one of my websites (www.immediateselfdefense.com for instance).

The introductory seminar may be enough for you. You may wish to repeat it every year or every couple of years to make sure the concepts really stick (the ideal would be to do it at least twice in the first year, and then periodically thereafter). This is what I imagine would be appropriate for most people, and would give them such a huge advantage, that it might meet all their Self Defense needs in life.

After the initial introductory seminar, however, you may wish to consider an intensive training weekend. On those weekends, we go for 2 or 3 days deeply into more difficult concepts. To me, the best training is when you do several intensive days with the same group of people. In order to be eligible for this training, there is an application and interview process, and candidates must pass a background check. (This may seem extreme, but I won't train just anyone, and when it comes to safety of my participants and students, I don't mess around.)

There are some amazing things that happen in intensive training situations that might take much longer in a conventional setting. As you train more, you get to know each other better, trust each other more, and it becomes safer for you to learn advanced concepts under pressure and with the effects of adrenaline. For everyone's safety, I always retain the option of uninviting anyone from the training before and during. If someone is not working in a constructive way, or they are out to cause injury instead of in it to learn, then I will not train them. Everyone's safety and a proper learning environment are my primary concerns.

If you are interested in learning some of my traditional Martial Arts in seminars, that is also a possibility. I have done some teaching of those curriculums in seminars, and would be open to doing more. To make it worth our mutual investments of time and money, and especially if there is much travel involved, I usually do an intensive training weekend, or at least a full day. I am open to teaching anything that I have learned to the right people. This might be appropriate for you if you have no experience whatsoever, but it might also be perfect if you have a ton of experience and would like to see a different perspective. I have found training like this to be incredibly valuable.

I especially enjoy working on the functional drills, training exercises, and techniques preserved in the ancient forms, for both weapons and empty hands. These were preserved by martial artists who devoted their lives to the study, and we would do well to honor them by practicing every part that they have left us.

Private Instruction

Practicing in groups is extremely valuable. I have always enjoyed practicing in groups. There is also a very wonderful energy that a group of people can develop together, working hard, being a team, cooperating towards a common goal, support for each other, and many more benefits. In groups, you get to work with people of all different shapes and sizes, and that's what it takes to get really proficient. Lots of practice with lots of different people, the more the better. Actually, that's a big part of the reason that I started teaching. I wanted to be good, and my teacher told me that by working with lots and lots of different people, I would be much better than if I didn't. Now I teach because I love it.

As valuable as practicing in groups is, private instruction is the perfect complement to it. When you learn privately or in very small groups, you can get very specific instruction, more hands-on time, and a level of detail and attention that is impossible to compare to only group instruction. In addition to regular group classes, I have always taken private lessons.

With a one on one private lesson, your teacher can get to know exactly what you know and show you exactly what you need to get better in a very profound way. When they are watching only you, and looking at everything you do, they will identify lots and lots of small details that you can improve. They can design training programs that will improve your specific trouble areas. They can adjust any exercises or skills that are not appropriate for your body, or give you a series of steps to accomplish your goals in a smoother and easier way. A teacher has spent a huge amount of time to get where they are. Private lessons are the ideal way to get the most from your investment of time and money.

All great teachers love to teach great students. To be a great student, you come early or on time, prepared to learn, make sure you have recently reviewed everything you need to, and have studied what you are assigned to study (you may read great texts like the "Art of War" by SunZi and learn to apply those lessons to your daily life).

If your mentality is not right (for instance you are very heavily distracted by something and not able to put it behind you), your teacher very likely will have special exercises designed to focus your mind and body. Some of my most valuable lessons were when I was distracted, unfocused, or frustrated by life's events, and I got to learn how to regulate my emotions, how to focus my mind, and how to move forward with the rest of my day in a better mood and state of mind. Actually, I'm sure I use these parts of my training far more than Self Defense. The "internal" aspects of Martial Arts are many, profound, and deep. Remember, ancient cultures have trained warriors for thousands of years to be strong and capable leaders, and to defend others. These traditions are alive and well in the Martial Arts, and you would do well to study them. They can have profound benefits for your whole life. Check out www.leaderprinciples.com.

One of the things I make frequent use of is videoing my students. They show me something they are working on, I video it, and we look at it together. I then am able to show them what they are doing, and where they can improve. I teach them to see what I see.

In small group private lessons, you may get to do hands-on work with another person with the careful supervision of your instructor. This is ideal for your group, because the teacher can make so many adjustments easily by being able to watch from the side.

A balanced mix of group instruction, private lessons, and small group lessons is the ideal way to learn the Martial Arts. I hope that if you study, your instructor includes the mental, emotional, and psychological trainings that I've been privileged to receive. If they are not, ask for this training. They perhaps did not realize you were interested, and may have a lot to offer.

Weekend Hiring

Isn't it fun to go away for the weekend? You bet. I love it. Would you like me to come and teach you or your group for a weekend? I'd probably love to come.

What aspects of training interest you? If it's something I do well, I'm happy to come see you. Contact me, and let's work it out. I love to train all kinds of people, in all kinds of skills.

However, maybe you are interested in something that's really outside my wheelhouse. (Groundfighting for the cage, for instance.) Good news! I know lots of Martial Arts teachers. I am certain that I know someone who can teach you what you would like to know.

But couldn't you just go seek out those instructors yourself? Certainly! But since they don't know you, you'd be starting from the beginning of the relationship, and they may or may not want to work with you. The best way to work with the best people is to have an introduction.

What does it take to get an introduction? Well, we have to know each other a bit before I would risk my good name introducing you to someone else. I would need to check you out, and get to know what kind of person you are. I would need to come visit you and assess your current skill in whatever you were interested in, and make sure you know whatever pre-requisites might be appropriate before I refer you to another instructor (they would not like to have a student introduced to them who was not ready to learn what they have to teach). I'm happy to introduce the right people to the right people. Everyone wins. I build a better relationship with that teacher, and they get a great student who is eager and ready to learn.

Licensing in Immediate Self Defense

I have not yet licensed anyone to teach Immediate Self Defense. However, I have plans to start a licensing program. I have taught several thousand people Self Defense at this point. The majority of those that have taken my course have no experience whatsoever. Some have some experience, but vastly prefer what and how I teach. Those few who have lots of experience have appreciated my approach, and seen its value. I have yet to have a Self Defense student who did not feel that they benefitted tremendously from what I have to teach. Just the other day, a student in a workshop told me he had learned something from me that he had never seen before, and he had law enforcement and military special forces training! To me it was a normal thing, but he really valued it. A fresh perspective can be very useful.

Because of my experience reaching an audience that is very different than the majority of Martial Arts students, I think I have something special to offer the world. Absolutely everyone would benefit from studying Self Defense. My wife says I want to put a shield around the whole world to keep everyone safe, so you can imagine my joy when I saw the cover design that the artist came up with (a big shield). The great news is that people are happy to pay for what I know. And those that invest their money as well as their time, take it far more seriously, and get far more out of it. I get to do what I love and have spent my life working on, serve my community, and get paid too. What could be better?

If you are a Martial Arts instructor, who better to teach Self Defense in your community? If you are not already reaching corporations, your local college and other schools, business leaders and your general community, let me help you! A Martial Arts instructor already has the majority of the skills needed, no matter what their art. You just need to learn the ideal way to put it all together, make it enjoyable, easy to learn, and simplified enough that it will work for the average person without a lot of training. I can teach you my Immediate Self Defense system faster than you might think, and License you to continue to teach it. It can be a great way for you to serve your community, build rapport with people you might otherwise never interact with, and has led me to be honored for service by my city.

Helping Martial Arts Teachers

I have met some tremendous Martial Arts teachers that would benefit from a little guidance. Sometimes even if you are a really good cook, someone else can still give you a few tips that will help you dramatically improve your recipe. This is why I have and honor mentors and teachers. Actually, everyone can teach you something if you are open to it.

I would like to help Martial Arts teachers. You might be very dedicated and excellent, but you might benefit from an outside objective look. You might be missing certain key things that you'd like to include in your curriculum, but are not getting the help you need from other sources. You might have learned primarily in group lessons and be missing those hundreds of little details that can make all the difference. You might just want to work with someone from a totally different source and with a very different perspective. I've worked with all kinds of different people, and always benefitted from it. Because of this, I have learned to respect all the arts and the teachers who dedicate themselves to training and teaching them.

It's a little awkward to offer this help because I am very young (in my early 40s), but I have dedicated my life to the study and training of Martial Arts, and I believe in service. If there is an opportunity for me to help you be a better Martial Arts teacher, and you are open to it, it would be my pleasure to serve. I'm sure I will benefit by working with you as much as you would by working with me.

The thing that I am best at is the application of classical forms, and the little details that make you more effective. Understanding the drills, concepts, theories, and training that is included in them for all teachers to work on for all time. I have an advantage in that the type of Kung Fu that I teach, 7 Star Praying Mantis Kung Fu from Mainland China, is incredibly intricate and detailed. Because my teacher had so many high level teachers himself, and I have so much extensive private training and small group training, I am able to see things from a very special perspective. It's really not that I'm special, it's that the skills that have been entrusted to me are precious, and it is my duty to share.

Joining our 501c3 Non-Profit

I founded a 501c3 non-profit Martial Arts school, Martial Arts Academy Bujutsu Gakuin Wushu Xueyuan. (Martial Arts Academy in English, Japanese, and Mandarin Chinese, because I teach arts from Japan, Okinawa, and China). It has been an amazing journey to start my own school, and I'm so honored that my teacher has supported and encouraged me to do so. He is now retired, and his wish is that I take what I have learned, and spread it far and wide in service to the ethics of Bushido of Japan and Wude of China (Ways of the Warrior/Scholar).

It's possible that you would like to join our organization and get ongoing support for your school. By collaborating, we might be even better than we could ever be individually. Obviously we would have to get to know each other well, and make sure that it would be a mutually beneficial relationship.

Other Collaborations

I hope that through this book, you have seen my sincere desire to serve through sharing what I know. If you can think of other ways that we can collaborate, I am very open to them. I am especially interested in making sure that all young ladies learn Self Defense, as all the studies show that ladies between the ages of 12-17 are the very most at risk, and then ladies age 25 and younger are the next most at risk. If every young lady could read this book, and get some hands-on Self Defense training, that could be a great start.

Maybe as you read this book, you would like to sell it to your own students, thinking that it complements your own Self Defense training courses. If it is useful to you, I would be honored! Please contact the publisher about special discounts for bulk purchases.

About the Author

The highly sought after instructor/author lives in the USA, in the Wine Country of Northern California, but loves to travel to conduct seminars and workshops on Self Defense, Martial Arts, and Leadership, to help business owners and professionals to know that they are safe, and to transform them into more effective Leaders.

Tony founded a 501c3 non-profit Martial Arts school, Martial Arts Academy 武術学院 Bujutsu Gakuin Wushu Xueyuan in Rohnert Park, California. Tony has been teaching Self Defense and Martial Arts professionally for more than a decade. He has studied several different disciplines of the Martial Arts for more than 20 years. He and his school have been awarded a Proclamation for Service to the City of Rohnert Park where his school is located.

He is a proud Rotarian, an organization devoted to "Service Above Self." As a Rotarian, Tony is proud to serve his community and the world with his knowledge of and love for Self Defense and Martial Arts and their many benefits. Not everyone has the time, interest, and devotion necessary for Martial Arts study, but Tony feels that EVERYONE needs to know Self Defense, and if you truly understood how this knowledge could change the lives of yourself and your loved ones, you would learn IMMEDIATELY.

With this book, he has shared his years of experience and unique concepts that have helped so many students to gain real confidence, and know that they are safe, and protect their loved ones.

For more information, see our websites:
www.theselfdefensebook.com
www.immediateselfdefense.com
www.martialartsacademy.online
www.leaderprinciples.com

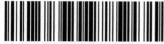

Made in the USA
San Bernardino, CA
19 August 2016